A Scoping Review of Clinical Studies About the Therapeutic Benefits of Medical Cannabis

Gabriel Bennett

A Scoping Review of Clinical Studies About the Therapeutic Benefits of Medical Cannabis

Springer

Gabriel Bennett
Independent Researcher
Klemzig, SA, Australia

ISBN 978-981-97-7940-6 ISBN 978-981-97-7941-3 (eBook)
https://doi.org/10.1007/978-981-97-7941-3

This Springer imprint is published by the registered company Springer Nature Singapore Pte Ltd.
The registered company address is: 152 Beach Road, #21-01/04 Gateway East, Singapore 189721, Singapore

Statement About the Usage of Artificial Intelligence

ChatGPT, a large language model artificial intelligence programme developed by the company OpenAI, was used to enhance the clarity of the concepts articulated in this book. All other procedures that were used to create this research was performed by Dr. Gabriel Bennett.

Contents

About the Author

Dr. Gabriel Bennett, Ph.D. the pen name for Dr. Matthew Bennett, holds a Ph.D. in Disability Studies from Flinders University, Australia. He has lectured in Disability Studies at Griffith University, Queensland. He has also advised the Australian Government's Autism CRC and has published articles for the *Journal of Autism and Developmental Disorders*. He is actively involved in supporting autistics and exploring key issues concerning disability. He has published several books, including:

Bennett, M., Webster, A. A., Goodall, E., & Rowland, S. (2019). *Life on the Autism Spectrum: Translating Myths and Misconceptions into Positive Futures*. Springer Nature. https://doi.org/10.1007/978-981-13-3359-0

Bennett, M., & Goodall, E. (2021). *Employment of Persons with Autism: A Scoping Review*. Springer Nature. https://doi.org/10.1007/978-3-030-82174-6

Bennett, M., & Goodall, E. (2022). *Addressing Underserved Populations in Autism Spectrum Research: An Intersectional Approach*. Emerald Publishing Group. https://doi.org/10.1108/9781803824635

Bennett, G. (2023). *Autistic People in Dental and Medical Clinics: Challenges and Solutions*. Springer Nature. https://doi.org/10.1007/978-981-99-2359-5

Acronyms

ADHD	Attention-Deficit Hyperactivity Disorder
AMA	Australian Medical Association
ARTG	Australian Register of Therapeutic Goods
CBMPs	Cannabis-Based Medicinal Products
CDSA	Controlled Drugs and Substances Act
GAD	Generalised Anxiety Disorder
GAD-7	General Anxiety Disorder-7
HRQoL	Health-Related Quality of Life
MMAR	Marihuana Medical Access Regulations
MMPR	Marihuana for Medical Purposes Regulations
PDS	Post-traumatic Diagnostic Scale
PRISMA	Preferred Reporting Items for Systematic Reviews and Meta-Analyses
PROMS	Patient-Reported Outcome Measures
PSQI-HQ	Pittsburgh Sleep Quality Index Hebrew version
PTSD	Post-traumatic Stress Disorder
RACGP	Royal Australian College of General Practitioners
SAS	Special Access Scheme
SQS	Sleep Quality Scale
TBI	Traumatic Brain Injury
TGA	Therapeutic Goods Administration
THC	Tetrahydrocannabinol
TS-CGI	Tourette Syndrome Clinical Global Impressions
TSSL	Tourette Syndrome Symptom List (patient rated)
YGTSS	Yale Global Tic Severity Scale

List of Figures

List of Tables

Chapter 1
Introduction

Abstract This chapter begins with an overview of medical cannabis laws in Australia, New Zealand, Canada, the United Kingdom, and the United States of America. The research questions that have guided this study and the rationale for these questions are then stated. In the following order, the search procedures for retrieving relevant citations, the methodological strengths and weaknesses of this study, the intended audience for this book, the benefits of this book, and a description of the upcoming chapters are then explained.

Keywords Health policy · Medical cannabis laws · Medical ethics · Methodological strengths and weaknesses · Recreational cannabis legalisation · Research questions · Search procedures · Special access scheme

1.1 Medical Cannabis Laws in the Anglosphere

1.1.1 Canada

Before 2001, seriously ill people in Canada had the option to appeal to the federal Minister of Health to be exempted from the *Controlled Drugs and Substances Act* (CDSA), which governed the use of substances like cannabis and opiates. This exemption, outlined in Section 56 of the CDSA, remained unused until Health Canada was directed by the Ontario Supreme Court to expand patient access to medical cannabis. Consequently, the Minister of Health granted permission, based on compassionate reasons, to two people living with acquired immunodeficiency syndrome to grow and consume their own cannabis (Shim et al., 2023).

However, these regulations were nullified by the courts in 2000. Terrance Parker, who had suffered from severe epilepsy since childhood, discovered that smoking cannabis was more effective than conventional medication in reducing his debilitating seizures. Despite lacking ministerial approval, he cultivated and used cannabis. In 1996, Parker faced charges under the CDSA. He succeeded in his trial, and when the crown appealed, the court ruled in Parker's favour once again. Additionally,

G. Bennett, *A Scoping Review of Clinical Studies About the Therapeutic Benefits of Medical Cannabis*, https://doi.org/10.1007/978-981-97-7941-3_1

the appeals court determined that the arbitrary nature of the Section 56 exemption violated patients' constitutional rights to life, liberty, and security (Shim et al., 2023).

Subsequently, Health Canada introduced the *Marihuana Medical Access Regulations* (MMAR) in 2001. Patients had to seek authorisation from Health Canada to possess cannabis. The application, spanning 29 pages, required various details, including written confirmation from the patient's primary physician (and in some cases, a specialist) demonstrating that the patient either received palliative care or experienced severe symptoms due to specific medical conditions or treatments, such as intense nausea from chemotherapy, which could not be alleviated with conventional pharmaceuticals. The initial patients were enrolled in the programme in early 2003 (Shim et al., 2023). Under the MMAR, people with authorisation or their representatives could acquire a permit to cultivate cannabis plants. Additionally, patients had the option to purchase dried cannabis from Health Canada at a rate of $5 per gram. These production licenses outlined the allowable number of cannabis plants, determined through a formula based on the authorised daily consumption and an estimated average yield per plant (Shim et al., 2023).

By December 2013, the average authorised daily consumption under the MMAR stood at approximately 18 g. People authorised for this daily intake were permitted to cultivate up to 88 cannabis plants. Delegated producers were able to grow cannabis on behalf of up to four authorised users, resulting in delegated production facilities potentially housing several hundred plants. Concerns arose among authorities regarding the safety implications of residential cannabis cultivation and the potential diversion of cannabis to the illegal market. These concerns were particularly significant in British Columbia, where more than two million cannabis plants were authorised under the MMAR (Shim et al., 2023).

In response to these concerns, Health Canada replaced the MMAR with the Marihuana for Medical Purposes Regulations (MMPR). Introduced in late 2013, and fully implemented by 1 April 2014, the MMPR revoked cannabis production licenses. Under these new regulations, authorised patients could solely obtain dried cannabis through mail order from licensed producers, commercial vendors regulated and approved by Health Canada (Shim et al., 2023).

The secondary objective of the MMPR was to remove Health Canada from the process of authorising patient access to medical cannabis. This responsibility was delegated to physicians and nurse practitioners, who could authorise cannabis use through a simplified one-page form referred to as a '*medical document*'. While Health Canada did not regulate cannabis potency or daily consumption, a possession limit of 150 g was established. To address the regulatory gaps, each provincial College of Physicians and Surgeons set its own prescribing limitations. These rules varied across provinces and included requirements for periodic patient consultations (every three months), risk assessments for addiction, and in Quebec enrolment in a cannabis use research study. Notably, authorities regulating nurse practitioners have not permitted cannabis prescribing (Shim et al., 2023).

Patient advocacy groups successfully lobbied the courts, resulting in landmark decisions allowing for the sale of cannabis oil and fresh cannabis leaves in 2015. Subsequently, patients or their representatives regained the right to cultivate cannabis

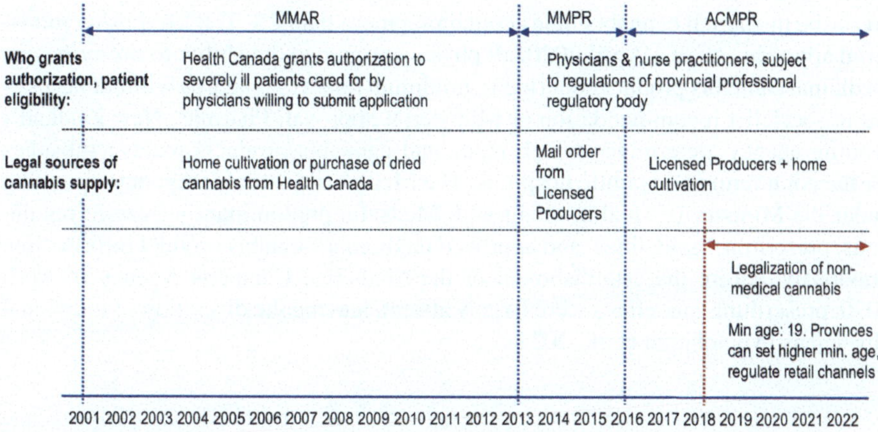

Fig. 1.1 Timeline of medical and recreational cannabis access regimes in Canada from 2001 to 2022. *MMAR* Marihuana medical access regulations; *MMPR* Marihuana for medical purposes regulations; *ACMPR* Access to cannabis for medical purposes regulations. *Source* Shim et al. (2023, p. 5)

for personal use in August 2016, albeit under more stringent regulations compared to the MMAR. These revised regulations are recognised as the *Access to Cannabis for Medical Purposes Regulations* (Shim et al., 2023).

In a more recent development, Canada made strides by legalising the recreational use of cannabis for people aged 19 or older in October 2018, making it only the second country, following Uruguay, to take this step. Like the previous regulations, only licensed producers are authorised to commercially cultivate cannabis, although people have the allowance to grow a limited number of cannabis plants for personal use. Each province exercises jurisdiction over various aspects, including cannabis usage regulations, such as age limitations for users and designated consumption areas, retail sales structures, imposition of excise taxes on cannabis sales, and the governance of personal cultivation. Recreational cannabis transactions are subject to federal and provincial excise taxes as well as sales taxes. Notably controversial, these taxes are also applicable to medical cannabis usage (Shim et al., 2023). Figure 1.1 provides an overview of the chronological sequence of medical and non-medical cannabis access regulations in Canada from 2001 to 2022.

1.1.2 New Zealand

Before April 2020, New Zealand's regulations concerning medicinal cannabis restricted general practitioners to prescribing Cannabidiol products with less than 2% Tetrahydrocannabinol (THC). Only specialised physicians had the authority to prescribe medicinal cannabis items containing more than 2% THC, requiring ministerial approval. As of 1 April 2020, all physicians gained the ability to prescribe any medicinal cannabis product adhering to minimum quality standards without necessitating specialist recommendation or Ministerial approval. Pharmac, New Zealand's funding agency, determines which medicinal cannabis products receive subsidies for the community and public hospitals. The Medicinal Cannabis Agency, operating under the Ministry of Health, along with Medsafe, predominantly oversee regulations, prescribing guidelines, and approved medicinal cannabis product information. Previously, before the establishment of the Medicinal Cannabis Agency in April 2020, prescribing guidelines were largely absent, leaving the discretion of individual physicians (Manoharan et al., 2022).

1.1.3 Australia

The Australian Government sanctioned the use of medicinal cannabis for specific therapeutic purposes on 1 November 2016. This legalisation facilitated the production and prescription of medicinal cannabis for therapeutic and research uses. However, most of these products are not listed on the Australian Register of Therapeutic Goods (ARTG). As a result, registered health practitioners must seek Therapeutic Goods Administration (TGA) approval before prescribing medicinal cannabis to their patients. TGA approval is typically determined on a case-by-case basis, contingent upon the specific conditions for which the medicinal cannabis is being prescribed (Hallinan & Bonomo, 2022).

Initially, the pathways for prescribing and accessing medicinal cannabis products across Australian State and Territory jurisdictions lacked uniformity. There existed a fragmented process for prescribing medicinal cannabis, requiring prescribers not only to understand how to prescribe within their local jurisdiction but also to justify their prescription. This convoluted and time-consuming process necessitated prescribers to submit paper-based applications to both the TGA and their respective state-based departments for prescription approval (Hallinan & Bonomo, 2022).

In July 2018, a centralised national online portal for medicinal cannabis prescription approval was introduced. This electronic platform allowed prescribers to electronically submit a single application directly to the TGA for prescription approval. Most jurisdictions, excluding Tasmania, embraced this national online system. Tasmania continued its independent management of cannabis prescribing through its Controlled Access Scheme, maintaining a state-based approval process. However, TGA approval statistics revealed substantially lower rates of medicinal cannabis prescribing per capita in Tasmania compared to other States and Territories (Hallinan & Bonomo, 2022).

Authorised medical cannabis prescribers, include Authorised Prescribers and Special Access Scheme (SAS) prescribers, secure approval for the use of medical cannabis via the Authorised Prescriber System or TGA SAS pathways. The Authorised Prescriber status is granted after medical practitioners apply to the TGA,

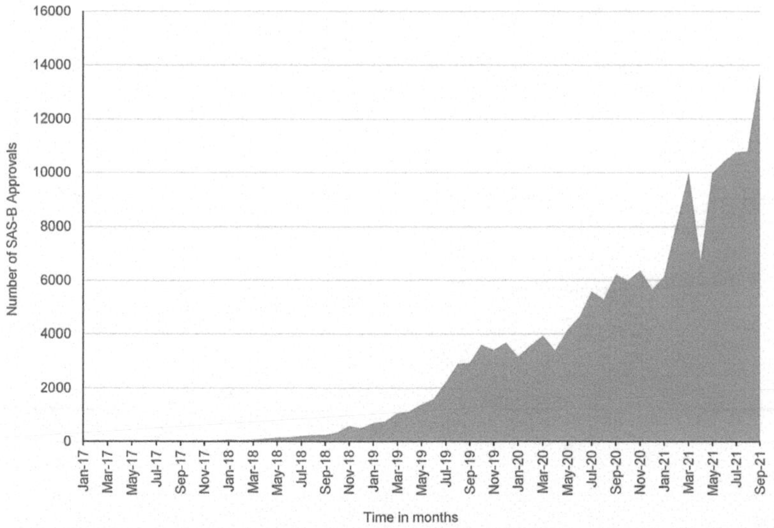

Fig. 1.2 Number of therapeutic goods administration (TGA) special access scheme category B (SAS-B) approvals monthly, from January 2017 to September 2021. *Notes* Adapted from TGA. Medicinal cannabis: role of the TGA Canberra, Australia: Department of Health Australia. *Source* Sabmeethavorn et al. (2022, p. 206)

allowing them to directly prescribe medicinal cannabis to their patients using an Authorised Prescriber script. Conversely, SAS prescribers must seek approval via an online TGA SAS application before providing a prescription to their patient. The SAS pathway consists of two main application categories: SAS-A providing an expedited pathway for prescribing to seriously ill patients and SAS-B catering to registered clinicians for multiple clinical indications. SAS-B application details include prescriber information, patient particulars, product type, and reasons for prescription. TGA SAS application approval can take up to 48 hours or more (Hallinan & Bonomo, 2022). Since its inception each year, there has been a systematic increase in the number of SAS-B prescriptions (see Fig. 1.2) This increase has been witnessed for various medical and psychological conditions and disabilities (see Fig. 1.3) (Cairns et al., 2023).

1.1.4 The United Kingdom of Great Britain and Northern Ireland

In the United Kingdom, there has long been a recognition that cannabis could be a legitimate medicinal option. However, despite numerous efforts urging the government to reconsider, the policy landscape had remained largely unchanged until recently. The turning point arrived in 2018 with two high-profile cases involving

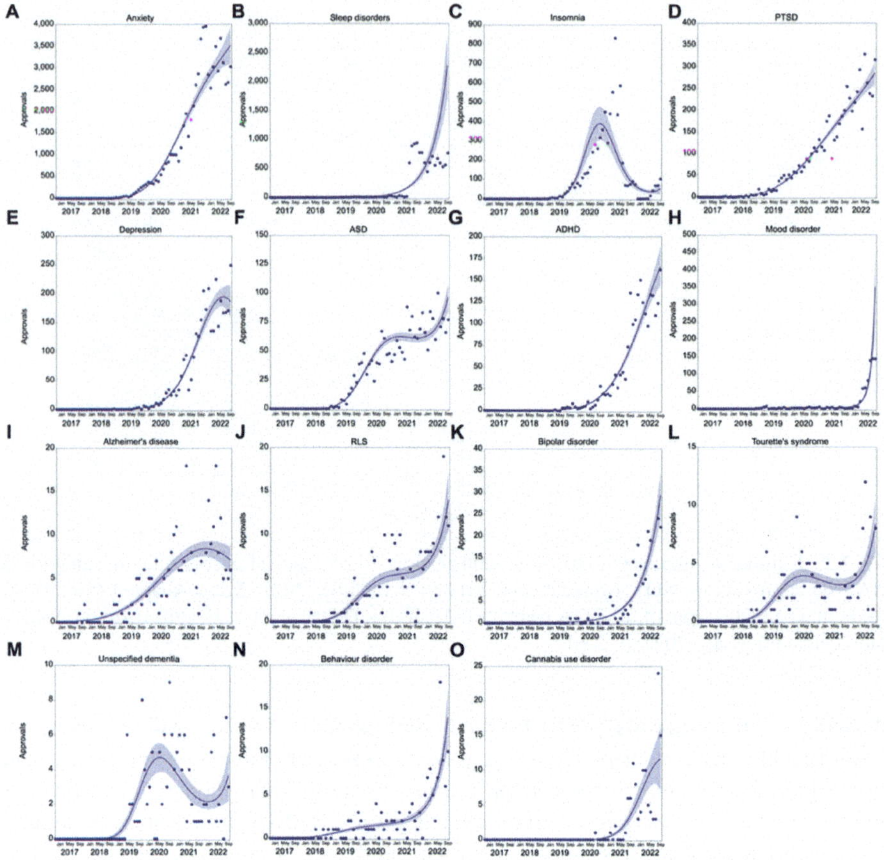

Fig. 1.3 Approvals per month in psychiatric indications with > 100 approvals. *Notes* Approvals over time for anxiety [**a**, n = 67,095]; sleep disorder [**b**, n = 11,202)], insomnia [**c**, n = 6877); post-traumatic stress disorder [PTSD; **d**, n = 5799]; depression [**e**, n = 3247]; autism spectrum disorder [ASD; **f**, n = 2206]; attention-deficit hyperactivity disorder [ADHD; **g**, n = 2078]; mood disorder [**h**, n = 736]; Alzheimer's disease [**i**, n = 272]; restless leg syndrome [RLS; **j**, n = 239]; bipolar disorder [**k**, n = 212]; Tourette's syndrome [**l**, n = 163]; unspecified dementia [**m**, n = 132]; behaviour disorder [**n**, n = 131]; cannabis use disorder [**o**, n = 117]. Solid lines represent the best fit, with shading depicting standard error of the mean (SEM). *Source* Cairns et al. (2023, p.10)

cannabis-based medicines used to treat severely ill children (i.e., Alfie Dingley and Billy Caldwell) who suffered from rare forms of epilepsy. This led to swift legislative changes, yet progress slowed amid the intricacies of evidence-based policymaking, decisions regarding medicines licensing, and the creation of clinical guidelines (Monaghan et al., 2021).

The Misuse of Drugs Act 1971 establishes the legal structure for governing dangerous or harmful drugs throughout the United Kingdom. This legislation categorises controlled substances into three classes based on their perceived risks and relative harm, with Class A considered the most harmful and Class C the least harmful. Presently, cannabis is classified under Class B, thereby carrying a maximum penalty of five-year imprisonment (with a possible fine) for possession and up to 14 years if there is an intent to supply. However, in practice, these maximum penalties are seldom imposed. Instances of possession without the intent to supply are typically addressed through alternative measures, such as cannabis warnings or on-the-spot fines. In conjunction with the Misuse of Drugs Act 1971, the Misuse of Drugs Regulations 2001 outlines the guidelines for lawful possession, supply, manufacturing, import, and export of substances prohibited by the Act. These regulations categorise substances into Schedules, ranging from Schedule 1 (i.e., containing drugs subject to stringent controls) to Schedule 5 (i.e., listing drugs exempt from most control requirements). Historically, cannabis has been classified under Schedule 1, grouped with other substances perceived to lack therapeutic value. Due to this classification, possessing or prescribing cannabis is not lawful (Monaghan et al., 2021).

Since 2001, there have been periodic revisions to the Misuse of Drugs Regulations. For example, Sativex, a cannabis-based medicine spray, is a Schedule 4 drug due to its acknowledged efficacy in treating multiple sclerosis-related spasticity. However, it remains an exception as a cannabis-based medicinal product within this classification. The legal framework for regulating '*cannabis-based products for medicinal use in humans*' is established by the 2018 Misuse of Drugs Regulations Amendment and the 2012 Human Medicines Regulations. Notably, on 1 November 2018 substances fitting the definition of cannabis-derived medicinal products, though the interpretation remains debatable, were reclassified from Schedule 1 to Schedule 2. This reclassification signifies that these products can now be prescribed and legally possessed with a valid prescription or authorisation (see Appendix A) (Monaghan et al., 2021).

1.1.5 The United States of America

In the nineteenth and early twentieth centuries, cannabis was widely used as a medicinal product in the United States of America and was officially recognised in the United States Pharmacopoeia in 1850. However, federal regulations on its usage and sale began in 1937 through the Marihuana Tax Act. Subsequently, cannabis was removed from the United States Pharmacopoeia in 1942, and stricter penalties for possession were imposed in 1951 and 1956 with the Boggs and Narcotic Control Acts. The Controlled Substances Act of 1970 federally prohibited cannabis. These legislative measures not only criminalised cannabis but also limited its research due to constraints on procurement for academic purposes. The Compassionate Use Act of 1996 in California marked the first state legalisation for medicinal cannabis under physician supervision. By 1 January 2017, 28 states along with Washington D.C., Guam, and Puerto Rico had enacted laws governing the sale and distribution of medicinal cannabis. Additionally, 21 states and Washington D.C. had decriminalised marijuana for possession of small amounts, while eight states (i.e., Alaska,

California, Colorado, Maine, Massachusetts, Nevada, Oregon, and Washington) and Washington D.C. had legalised marijuana for adult recreational use (Bridgeman & Abazia, 2017).

1.2 Research Questions

A comparison of the legalisation status of medical/medicinal cannabis within different nations in the anglosphere has revealed several common trends. First, at different rates, each nation is changing its laws to give medical staff the option to prescribe medicinal/medical cannabis to patients who meet certain access requirements. Second, due to its legalisation, the amount of research about the therapeutic benefits of medicinal/medical cannabis for different disabilities, as well as different medical and psychological conditions, is increasing. Third, with the legalisation of medicinal/medical cannabis, the opportunity to ask patients and medical personnel about their experiences with this medication has emerged. In the interests of improving our understanding about the clinical benefits and drawbacks of medicinal/medical cannabis and the enablers and barriers of prescribing this medication the following two research questions guided this study:

- Since 30 December 2018 to 30 December 2023 what are the findings in the literature about the benefits and drawbacks of using medicinal/medical cannabis to treat disabilities, medical conditions, and psychological conditions?
- Since 30 December 2018 to 30 December 2023 what are the findings in the literature about the views of clinicians, general practitioners, patients, and pharmacists about medicinal/medical cannabis?

1.3 Search Procedures for Relevant Citations

On 7 January 2024, a search of PubMed was conducted to retrieve citations that could answer the research questions. It was possible to search individual academic publishers (e.g., Routledge, Springer Nature, and SAGE). However, this approach was deemed to be ineffective because it would have involved a duplication of search procedures. Consequently, opting for a PubMed search was deemed more effective in identifying relevant references to address the research questions. This decision was motivated by two key factors. First, PubMed contained citations from various academic publishers, enabling the retrieval of references through a single search. Second, PubMed includes articles from academic publishers that the researcher might not have been aware of, facilitating the identification of relevant studies that would not have been anticipated through individual searches by the researcher.

A *Preferred Reporting Items for Systematic Reviews and Meta-Analyses* (PRISMA) approach was used to search and examine the citations retrieved from

PubMed. PRISMA is an established and widely used approach for collecting, examining, and identifying studies that answer a study's predetermined research questions from a large sample of retrieved literature. The PRISMA approach has five steps. These five steps and their relation to this study are listed below.

- STEP ONE: The first step was searching PubMed for studies about medicinal/medical cannabis for people with disabilities, medical, or psychological conditions. The search phrases (‘*medicinal cannabis*’ [Title]) OR (‘*medical cannabis*’ [Title]) were used to retrieve studies.
- STEP TWO: The second step involved removing any duplicate records that were retrieved from the single search of PubMed. No duplicate records were identified.
- STEP THREE: The third step involved examining each study's title and abstract to determine whether it met the study's eligibility criteria. To be included in this study, the citation had to have:

  – a sample of participants with disabilities and/or professionals who assist participants with disabilities,
  – been published in English, and
  – been published between 30 December 2018 and 30 December 2023.

The citation could also be a literature review or a meta-analysis. However, citations that were retractions, corrections, letters to the editor, or commentaries were excluded from this study.

Of the 683 studies that were retrieved from the first step, 79 were deemed to be of interest.

- STEP FOUR: The fourth step involved reading the entire text of the 79 studies that were provisionally deemed to answer one or both research questions. However, 20 studies could not be retrieved because they required payment to access. Of the 59 studies that could be accessed and examined, 10 were deemed to not answer one or both research questions.
- STEP FIVE: The fifth and final step involved summarising and explaining the results from the 49 studies that were retained from the fourth step in the PRISMA analysis process (see Fig. 1.4).

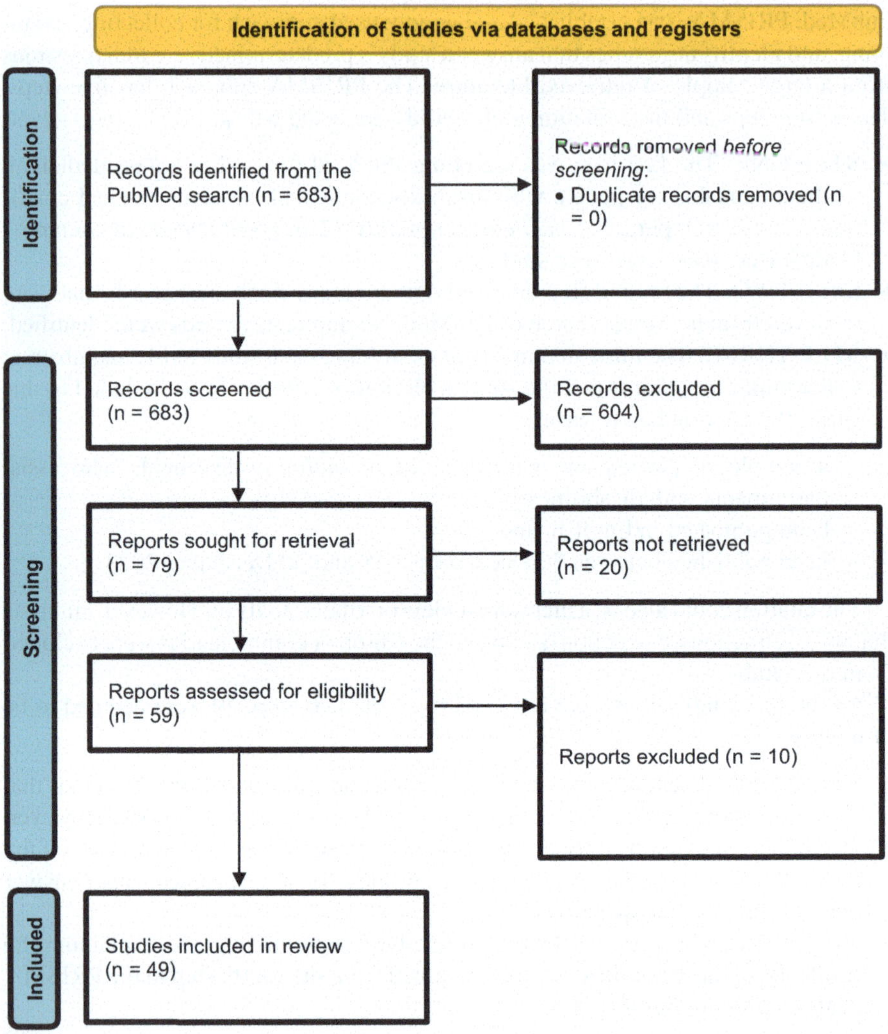

Fig. 1.4 Preferred reporting items for systematic reviews and meta-analyses (PRISMA) flow diagram. *Source* Page et al. (2021)

1.4 Methodological Strengths and Weaknesses of This Study

1.4.1 Methodological Strengths

1.4.1.1 Publication of the Study's Dataset

The inability to repeat a study because its methodology is inadequately described and/or the dataset was not published along with the study has been termed the *'reproducibility crisis'*. To avoid this book contributing to this crisis, this study's dataset is included as an appendix and the methodology for examining the dataset is clearly and adequately described (see Appendix B).

1.4.2 Methodological Weaknesses

1.4.2.1 Only Accessing Studies from PubMed

All studies reviewed in this book were sourced from a single search of PubMed on 7 January 2024. PubMed was used because it was deemed to be one of the largest repositories of English-language medical literature. Despite its size, not all studies about medical/medicinal cannabis are located on this database. Thus, there are studies that were not discovered and presented because their citations were not stored on PubMed. However, considering that many studies were recovered from PubMed, there was no need to search other repositories of medical literature.

1.4.2.2 Restricting the Search Terms to the Article's Title

To ensure that the maximum number of studies were retrieved, the search phrases *'medical cannabis'* and *'medicinal cannabis'* were used to retrieve studies that contained these terms in the citation's title. This approach was used because a considerable number of citations were retrieved when a search of the citation's abstract using these search phrases was conducted.

1.4.2.3 Only Examining English-Language Studies

In this book, only studies published in English were examined because this was the researcher's native language. Thus, insights from studies that were not published in English were not examined. However, this limitation was deemed as inconsequential because enough studies about the experiences of patients and healthcare professionals either prescribing or taking medical/medicinal cannabis were identified and analysed.

1.4.2.4 Only Examining Studies with Participants

To be included in this book, the study had to have had a sample of participants and been peer reviewed. Consequently, preprinted articles, letters to the editor, and other publications that did not contain samples of participants were not examined (Syed et al., 2023a, 2023b). Due to their omission, potentially valuable insights that could have contributed to the conclusions of this study were not examined.

1.5 Intended Audience of This Book

This book has been written for many different audiences, including:

- *Researchers and Academics:* This audience includes scientists, medical professionals, pharmacologists, and researchers who are interested in the field of medical cannabis and its therapeutic applications. This book can provide them with a comprehensive overview of existing clinical studies, helping them stay updated with the latest research in the field.
- *Healthcare Professionals:* This audience comprises doctors, nurses, and other healthcare practitioners who may be interested in understanding the potential therapeutic benefits of medical cannabis for their patients. This book can provide them with evidence-based information to support their clinical decision-making.
- *Policy Makers and Regulators:* Government officials, policymakers, and individuals involved in shaping healthcare policies would find this book valuable in understanding the scientific evidence behind medical cannabis. It can help them make informed decisions about regulations, legislation, and the integration of medical cannabis into healthcare systems.
- *Pharmaceutical Industry Professionals:* People working in the pharmaceutical industry, including drug development, research, and marketing, may be interested in exploring the potential therapeutic uses of cannabis-derived compounds. This book can serve as a reference for them to understand the current state of research in this field.
- *Patients and General Public:* People who are considering or currently using medical cannabis as a treatment option would benefit from this book. It can provide them with an in-depth understanding of the therapeutic benefits, potential risks, and limitations of medical cannabis based on scientific evidence.

1.6 Benefits of This Book

This book will provide many benefits for the reader, including:

- *Comprehensive Scoping Review:* This book offers a comprehensive scoping review of clinical studies, presenting a wide range of evidence on the therapeutic benefits of medical cannabis. It consolidates and synthesises findings from diverse sources, providing readers with a holistic understanding of the current state of knowledge.
- *Evidence-Based Approach:* The book emphasises an evidence-based approach, focussing on clinical studies that have evaluated the efficacy and safety of medical cannabis. By presenting the latest scientific evidence, readers can make informed decisions and gain confidence in the therapeutic potential of medical cannabis.
- *Broad Spectrum of Medical Conditions:* Unlike other literature, this book explores the therapeutic benefits of medical cannabis across a broad spectrum of medical conditions. It covers chronic pain, epilepsy, multiple sclerosis, cancer-related symptoms, and mental health disorders, making it a valuable resource for healthcare professionals and patients seeking treatment options.
- *User-Friendly Organisation:* The book is thoughtfully organised, making it easy for readers to navigate and locate specific information. It provides clear sections on each medical condition, allowing readers to quickly access relevant studies, findings, and recommendations.
- *Timely and Relevant:* Given the increasing interest and evolving legal landscape surrounding medical cannabis, this book addresses a timely and relevant topic. It provides up-to-date information on the therapeutic potential of medical cannabis, making it an essential resource for researchers, healthcare professionals, policymakers, and individuals seeking alternative treatment options.

These points highlight the uniqueness of this book and demonstrate why it is likely to appeal to, and be purchased by, the core audience of readers interested in exploring the therapeutic benefits of medical cannabis.

1.7 Description of Upcoming Chapters

1.7.1 Chapter Two—Benefits and Drawbacks of Patients Using Cannabis

Within Chapter two, the therapeutic benefits and drawbacks of patients using medical/medicinal cannabis for various medical conditions, disabilities, and psychological conditions are presented. The purpose of presenting these results is to inform the reader about utility of medical/medicinal cannabis for various conditions.

1.7.2 Chapter Three—Views Among Healthcare Professionals and Patients About Medical Cannabis

The results in the retrieved literature about the experiences and views of healthcare professionals prescribing medical/medicinal cannabis are presented in Chapter three. This chapter will help the reader understand the barriers that healthcare professionals encounter when prescribing medical/medicinal cannabis, such as not know knowing the potential therapeutic benefits of this medication for specific conditions or not knowing the regulatory framework for legally prescribing medical/medicinal cannabis.

1.7.3 Chapter Four—Future Research Directions and Closing Remarks

The final chapter of this book summarises the gaps in our existing literature. The purpose of this chapter is to present an overview of this field of research.

1.8 Additional Readings

1.8.1 National Policies

1.8.1.1 Canada

Armstrong M. J. (2023). Relationships between sales of legal medical cannabis and alcohol in Canada. *Health policy (Amsterdam, Netherlands)*, *128*, 28–33. https://doi.org/10.1016/j.healthpol.2022.11.012

Awal, M., Kelly, L. E., Anderson, J., Brace, T., Brown, C., Buettner, T., King, P. M., Klemmer, J., Lougheed, T., O'Shea, K., & Mansell, H. (2022). Medical Cannabis in Canadian Schools: A Scoping Review of Existing Policies. *Cannabis and Cannabinoid Research*, *7*(6), 758–768. https://doi.org/10.1089/can.2021.0199

Carnide, N., Lee, H., Landsman, V., Frone, M. R., Furlan, A. D., & Smith, P. M. (2022). Cannabis use and workplace cannabis availability, perceptions and policies among Canadian workers: a comparison before and after the legalisation of non-medical cannabis. *Occupational and Environmental Medicine*, *79*(12), 824–830. https://doi.org/10.1136/oemed-2022-108316

Myran, D. T., Friesen, E. L., Dickson, S., Konikoff, L., Arora, G., & Tanuseputro, P. (2023). Access to legal cannabis market in Canada over the four years following non-medical cannabis legalisation. *Drug and Alcohol Review*, *42*(5), 1114–1119. https://doi.org/10.1111/dar.13650

Nguyen, H. V., Grootendorst, P., Mital, S., Bishop, L., & McGinty, E. E. (2024). Changes in Medical Cannabis Use After Recreational Cannabis Legalization in Canada. *Cannabis and Cannabinoid Research*, *9*(1), 335–342. https://doi.org/10.1089/can.2022.0227

Shim, M., Nguyen, H., & Grootendorst, P. (2023). Lessons from 20 years of medical cannabis use in Canada. *PloS One*, *18*(3), e0271079. https://doi.org/10.1371/journal.pone.0271079

1.8.1.2 Australia

Erku, D., Greenwood, L. M., Graham, M., Hallinan, C. M., Bartschi, J. G., Renaud, E., & Scuffham, P. (2022). From growers to patients: Multi-stakeholder views on the use of, and access to medicinal cannabis in Australia. *PloS One*, *17*(11), e0277355. https://doi.org/10.1371/journal.pone.0277355

Graham, M., Chiu, V., Stjepanović, D., & Hall, W. (2023). A provisional evaluation of Australia's medical cannabis program. *The International Journal on Drug Policy*, *122*, 104210. https://doi.org/10.1016/j.drugpo.2023.104210

Hallinan, C. M., & Bonomo, Y. A. (2022). The Rise and Rise of Medicinal Cannabis, What Now? Medicinal Cannabis Prescribing in Australia 2017-2022. *International Journal of Environmental Research and Public Health*, *19*(16), 9853. https://doi.org/10.3390/ijerph19169853

MacPhail, S. L., Bedoya-Pérez, M. A., Cohen, R., Kotsirilos, V., McGregor, I. S., & Cairns, E. A. (2022). Medicinal Cannabis Prescribing in Australia: An Analysis of Trends Over the First Five Years. *Frontiers in Pharmacology*, *13*, 885655. https://doi.org/10.3389/fphar.2022.885655

1.8.1.3 United Kingdom

Erridge, S., Coomber, R., & Sodergren, M. H. (2022). Medical cannabis, CBD wellness products and public awareness of evolving regulations in the United Kingdom. *Journal of Cannabis Research*, *4*(1), 56. https://doi.org/10.1186/s42238-022-00165-6

1.8.1.4 New Zealand

Withanarachchie, V., Rychert, M., & Wilkins, C. (2023). Barriers and facilitators to prescribing medicinal cannabis in New Zealand. *Journal of Primary Health Care*, *15*(2), 135–146. https://doi.org/10.1071/HC22122

1.8.1.5 United States of America

Hong, G., Sideris, A., Waldman, S., Stauffer, J., & Wu, C. L. (2024). Legal and Regulatory Aspects of Medical Cannabis in the United States. *Anesthesia and Analgesia, 138*(1), 31–41. https://doi.org/10.1213/ANE.0000000000006301

References

Bridgeman, M. B., & Abazia, D. T. (2017). Medicinal cannabis: History, pharmacology, and implications for the acute care setting. *P & t: A Peer-Reviewed Journal for Formulary Management, 42*(3), 180–188.

Cairns, E. A., Benson, M. J., Bedoya-Pérez, M. A., Macphail, S. L., Mohan, A., Cohen, R., Sachdev, P. S., & McGregor, I. S. (2023). Medicinal cannabis for psychiatry-related conditions: An overview of current Australian prescribing. *Frontiers in Pharmacology, 14*, 1142680. https://doi.org/10.3389/fphar.2023.1142680

Hallinan, C. M., & Bonomo, Y. A. (2022). The rise and rise of medicinal cannabis, what now? Medicinal cannabis prescribing in Australia 2017–2022. *International Journal of Environmental Research and Public Health, 19*(16), 9853. https://doi.org/10.3390/ijerph19169853

Manoharan, R., Kemper, J., & Young, J. (2022). Exploring the medical cannabis prescribing behaviours of New Zealand physicians. *Drug and Alcohol Review, 41*(6), 1355–1366. https://doi.org/10.1111/dar.13476

Monaghan, M., Wincup, E., & Hamilton, I. (2021). Scandalous decisions: Explaining shifts in UK medicinal cannabis policy. *Addiction (Abingdon, England), 116*(7), 1925–1933. https://doi.org/10.1111/add.15350

Page, M. J., McKenzie, J. E., Bossuyt, P. M., Boutron, I., Hoffmann, T. C., Mulrow, C. D., Shamseer, L., Tetzlaff, J. M., Akl, E. A., Brennan, S. E., Chou, R., Glanville, J., Grimshaw, J. M., Hróbjartsson, A., Lalu, M. M., Li, T., Loder, E. W., Mayo-Wilson, E., McDonald, S., McGuinness, L. A., et al. (2021). The PRISMA 2020 statement: An updated guideline for reporting systematic reviews. *BMJ (Clinical Research ed.), 372*,. https://doi.org/10.1136/bmj.n71

Sabmeethavorn, Q., Bonomo, Y. A., & Hallinan, C. M. (2022). Pharmacists' perceptions and experiences of medicinal cannabis dispensing: A narrative review with a systematic approach. *The International Journal of Pharmacy Practice, 30*(3), 204–214. https://doi.org/10.1093/ijpp/riac005

Shim, M., Nguyen, H., & Grootendorst, P. (2023). Lessons from 20 years of medical cannabis use in Canada. *PLoS ONE, 18*(3), e0271079. https://doi.org/10.1371/journal.pone.0271079

Syed, S. A., Singh, J., Elkholy, H., Palavra, I. R., Tomicevic, M., Eric, A. P., da Costa, M. P., Guloksuz, S., & Radhakrishnan, R. (2023a). International perspective on physician knowledge, attitude and practices related to medical cannabis. *medRxiv: The Preprint Server for Health Sciences*, 2023.07.26.23293157. https://doi.org/10.1101/2023.07.26.23293157

Syed, S. A., Singh, J., Elkholy, H., Rojnić Palavra, I., Tomicevic, M., Eric, A. P., Pinto da Costa, M., Guloksuz, S., & Radhakrishnan, R. (2023b). Impact of personal beliefs about medical cannabis on physician recommendation practices: Results of an international survey. *Asian Journal of Psychiatry, 85*, 103634. https://doi.org/10.1016/j.ajp.2023.103634

Chapter 2
Benefits and Drawbacks of Patients Using Cannabis

Abstract This chapter presents the results in the studies retrieved from the PubMed search that explain the therapeutic benefits and drawbacks that medical/medicinal cannabis can have on different disabilities, psychiatric and medical conditions. The conditions discussed in this chapter are anxiety, attention-deficit hyperactivity disorder, intellectual disabilities, Post-traumatic stress disorder, West syndrome, sleep disorders and insomnia, depression, treatment-resistant epilepsy, brain injury, autism spectrum disorders, multiple sclerosis, Parkinson's disease, and Gilles de la Tourette. This chapter will give readers an appreciation of the potential therapeutic benefits and drawbacks that medical/medicinal cannabis can give people with these conditions.

Keywords Anxiety · Attention-deficit hyperactivity disorder (ADHD) · Autism spectrum disorder · Brain injury · Depression · Gilles de la Tourette · Insomnia · Intellectual disabilities · Multiple sclerosis · Parkinson's disease · Post-traumatic stress disorder (PTSD) · Sleep disorders · Treatment-resistant epilepsy · West syndrome

2.1 Anxiety (Including Generalised Anxiety Disorder)

An examination of the 683 citations retrieved from the PubMed search yielded four studies that contained results about the therapeutic benefits that medical cannabis had on a person's anxiety (Bapir et al., 2023; Ergisi et al., 2022; Rifkin-Zybutz et al., 2023; Sachedina et al., 2022). The aims, methodologies, and results of these four studies are now presented.

Bapir et al. (2023) compared the therapeutic outcomes of patients with chronic pain who either did or did not have comorbid anxiety following the consumption of cannabis-based medicinal products (CBMPs). Before consuming CBMPs the participant's anxiety was measured using the General Anxiety Disorder-7 (GAD-7) test. Participants were divided into two groups; those who did not have anxiety (GAD-7 < 5) and those who did have anxiety (GAD-7 ≥ 5). Participants completed at one,

G. Bennett, *A Scoping Review of Clinical Studies About the Therapeutic Benefits of Medical Cannabis*, https://doi.org/10.1007/978-981-97-7941-3_2

three, and six months into the study the *Brief Pain Inventory Short-Form, Short-Form McGill Pain Questinnaire-2, Pain Visual Analogue Scale, Sleep Quality Scale, GAD-7*, and *EQ-5D-5L*. The scores from these testes were used to determine the primary outcomes of the study. In total, 1254 participants (anxiety $n = 711$, no anxiety $n = 543$) met the inclusion criteria. These researchers concluded that the consumption of CBMPs potentially relieved pain and improved health-related quality of life (HRQoL) among patients with chronic pain. Furthermore, patients with chronic pain and comorbid anxiety also reported greater improvements in HRQoL.

Ergisi et al. (2022) explored the therapeutic benefits of medicinal cannabis in treating people with generalised anxiety disorder (GAD). In total, 67 patients who attended the Sapphire Clinics for medicinal cannabis treatment for GAD participated in their study. Ergisi et al. reported that medicinal cannabis might improve GAD among patients, general health-related quality of life, and sleep-specific outcomes at one, three, and six months after they have begun taking medicinal cannabis.

Rifkin-Zybutz et al. (2023) evaluated the clinical outcomes of patients with GAD who were treated with dried flower, oil-based preparations, or a combination of both CBMPs. For their study, the primary outcomes were changes in GAD-7 questionnaire scores at one, three, and six months compared to GAD-7 scores collected at baseline. Additionally, secondary outcomes were single-item sleep quality scale (SQS) and health-related quality of life index (EQ-5D-5L) questionnaire scores that were taken at the same time points as the GAD-7 scores. Rifkin-Zybutz et al. reported that improvements in GAD symptoms, sleep quality, and quality of life were detected at each time point. In contrast, 39 participants (12.9%) reported 269 adverse events during the follow-up period. Similar developmental trends were also reported by Sachedina et al. (2022) and by the studies documented in Sarris et al.'s (2020) literature review (see Appendix C).

2.2 Attention-Deficit Hyperactivity Disorder (ADHD)

One study was discovered from the 683 citations retrieved from the PubMed search in which the therapeutic benefits of medical cannabis for people with attention-deficit hyperactivity disorder (ADHD) were measured (Ittiphakorn et al., 2023). Ittiphakorn et al. (2023) examined the impact on health-related quality of life (HRQoL) and safety that cannabis-based medicinal products (CBMPs) gave 68 people with ADHD. The UK Medical Cannabis Registry was used to source participants. Patient-reported outcomes from the EQ-5D-5L (i.e., the EQ-5D-5L was used to gauge HRQoL), generalised anxiety disorder (GAD-7), and the single-item Sleep Quality Score (SQS) were collected at baseline and at one, three, six, and 12 months from baseline. Data from these instruments formed the primary outcomes of the study. Participants' self-reported incidences of adverse events were the secondary outcomes assessed. Any statistical findings that were $p < 0.050$ were deemed statistically significant. They discovered that scores from the EQ-5D-5L improved over one, three, and six months; which denotes an improved HRQoL. Additionally, scores from the GAD-7 and SQS at one, three, six, and 12 months also showed that the participants generally had less anxiety and better quality of sleep. In contrast, 11 participants reported having an adverse event. In total, 61 adverse events were recorded, of which 19 were '*mild*', 26 were '*moderate*', and 16 were '*severe*'. Based on these results, Ittiphakorn et al. (2023, p. 602) concluded:

> This study reports that treatment with CBMPs was associated with improvements in general HRQoL [Health-Related Quality of Life] after 1, 3, and 6, months, in addition to anxiety and sleep quality after 1, 3, 6, and 12 months ($p<0.050$). These results suggest that CBMPs may play a role in alleviating symptoms and comorbid anxiety and sleep disruption associated with ADHD, though these are preliminary findings. CBMPs were well-tolerated throughout this study and the majority of patients (83.82%) did not report any adverse events. Due to limitations in study design, a causal relationship cannot be determined, thus, a definite conclusion cannot be drawn from these results.

2.3 Intellectual Disability

Out of the 683 citations that were retrieved from the PubMed search, one study by Korb et al. (2023) described the benefits that medicinal cannabis gave people with intellectual disability with managing their challenging behaviours. They reviewed six studies about the efficacy of medicinal cannabis for mental health and neurodevelopmental conditions (see Appendix D).

Based on the studies analysed, Korb et al. identified three practical challenges regarding researching the utility of medicinal cannabis in helping people with intellectual disabilities manage their challenging behaviours. First, there is a lack of research about adverse effects that people with intellectual disabilities experience after taking medicinal cannabis, such as withdrawal symptoms, potential for dependence, and interactions with other medicines. Second, participants with intellectual disability are often excluded from studies due to ethical concerns that they are unable to consent to being researched. Third, people with intellectual disabilities are not part of a homogeneous group because the severity of intellectual impairment and comorbidity profile varies between people with intellectual disabilities. Despite these limitations, Korb et al. (2023, p. 1206) concluded that:

> There remains a lack of effective psychosocial and pharmacological interventions for managing serious challenging behaviour in PwID [people with intellectual disabilities], which has significant implications on their quality of life, health and social outcomes. Too often, the research community has not been bold enough to insist that research is vital for the care of PwID. Using the complex issue of capacity to consent as an excuse not to progress research is simply not good enough. There is therefore the need to look for alternative, safer treatment approaches, principally to be used in combination with existing non-pharmacological management options. Medicinal cannabis particularly CBD appears to offer a potentially exciting new development, based on its reported therapeutic benefits for PwID in treating generalised anxiety disorder, as well as behavioural and psychological symptoms associated with dementia.

2.4 Post-traumatic Stress Disorder (PTSD)

Three studies were identified from the 683 citations retrieved from the PubMed search that contained results about the therapeutic benefits that medical/medicinal cannabis gives people with Post-traumatic stress disorder (PTSD) (Krediet et al., 2020; Nacasch et al., 2023; Pillai et al., 2022).

With the intention of acquiring patients' insights on and experiences with medical cannabis, Krediet et al. (2020) facilitated a focus group discussion among seven military veterans who were diagnosed with PTSD and who were using medical cannabis. After the focus group session, an evaluation was conducted, and during this evaluation, four partners of the veterans who were interviewed joined the group discussion. Both sessions were audio-recorded, transcribed verbatim, and analysed. The researchers identified five themes. Four of these five themes are related to the different phases of medical cannabis use—consideration, initiation, usage, and discontinuation. The fifth theme is related to several aspect of medicinal cannabis usage. For example, participants did not express a desire to use medicinal cannabis to '*get high*' but to instead manage their symptoms of PTSD. Additionally, participants explained that they had tried different strains and dosages of cannabis and reported several benefits, including better quality of sleep. Based on these results, Krediet et al. (2020, p. 251) concluded:

> Lack of therapeutic effect and/or experienced side effects with conventional medication played an important role in patients' decisions to consider cannabis as a potential treatment alternative. Patients expressed a wish to reduce or stop the use of other medications, and some reported having done so. They reported minimal side effects of medical cannabis and strongly favored it over many of the other medications that they had used in terms of the ratio of therapeutic effects to side effects. However, this general sentiment could have emerged due to the sample consisting of patients who had been dissatisfied with previous treatments.

Nacasch et al. (2023) measured the impact that medicinal cannabis had on the quality of sleep and PTSD symptoms of 14 veterans with PTSD. All participants completed the *Pittsburgh Sleep Quality Index Hebrew version* (PSQI-H) and the *Post-traumatic Diagnostic Scale* (PDS). Nacasch et al. only used part three of the PDS questionnaire, which was composed of 17 questions. These questions were designed to measure the severity/frequency of PTSD symptoms in the past month, and the responses ranged between 0 (i.e., never or once in the past two weeks) and 3 (i.e., at least five times a week). Regarding the PSQI-H, Nacasch et al. only used the following questions:

- subjective quality of sleep rated between 0 (very good) and 3 (very bad),
- duration of hours of sleep,
- inability to fall asleep within 30 min rated between 0 (not in the past month) and 3 (three or more times a week), and
- total score calculated from all ten questions (higher scores indicate worse sleep quality).

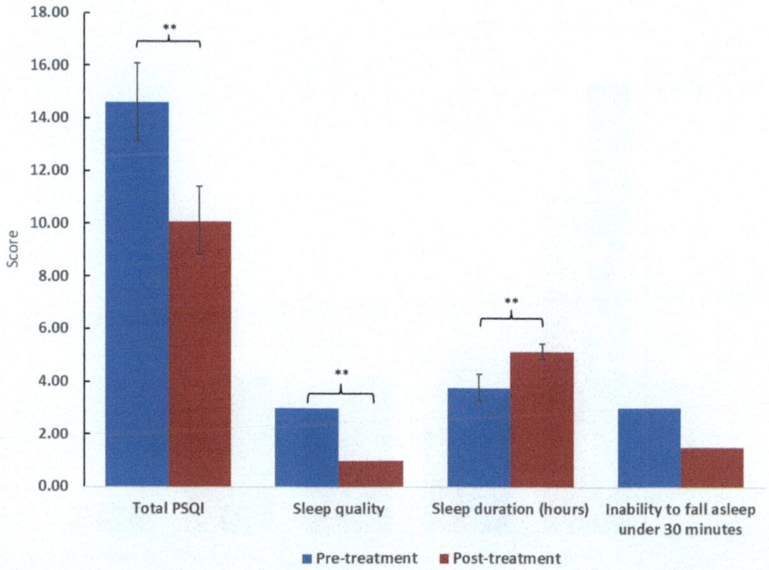

Fig. 2.1 Scores of post-traumatic diagnostic scale (PDS) and selected subdomains. *Notes* Higher scores reflect worse symptom severity. *Significance* $^{*}p < 0.05$, $^{**}p < 0.01$. For ratio and quasi-interval scales, means and standard errors are displayed, while medians are displayed for ordinal scales. *Source* Nacasch et al. (2023, p. 4)

Based on the data collected from the participants who completed these surveys, Nacasch et al. reported that the usage of medicinal cannabis improved sleep quality, total PSQI scores (see Fig. 2.1), and total PDS scores (see Fig. 2.2).

Pillai et al. (2022) measured the changes to HRQoL and any adverse events that patients with PTSD experienced while taking CBMPs. They examined 162 patient records that were sourced from the UK Medical Cannabis Registry. At time points one, three, and six months, they analysed HRQoL using patient-reported outcome measures. The *Common Terminology Criteria for Adverse Events version 4.0* was used to identify and analyse adverse events. Furthermore, statistical significance was defined as $p < 0.050$. Out of the 162 patient records examined, 144 (88.89%) were either current or previous cannabis users. Pillai et al. discovered that PTSD symptom reduction, improvements in sleep, and reductions in anxiety occurred over the three time points ($p < 0.050$). Additionally, 33 patients (20.37%) of the 162 patients examined reported adverse events. The severity of most of these events were classified as either *'mild'* or *'moderate'* ($n = 190$, 117.28%). Finally, most commonly occurring adverse events were insomnia and fatigue ($n = 20$, 12.35%). Similar results were reported by the studies examined by Sarris et al. (2020) (see Appendix C). Based on these findings, Pillai et al. (2022, p. 1016) concluded that:

> This observational study suggests an association between CBMP treatment and improvement in PTSD-specific, HRQoL, sleep, and anxiety outcomes at up to 6-month follow-up (p < 0.050). Treatment safety assessed via AE incidence demonstrated minimal severity and

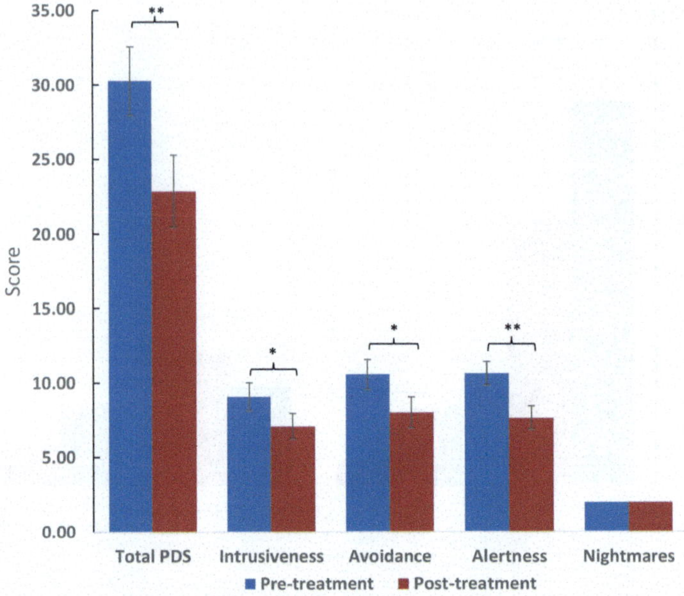

Fig. 2.2 Scores of Pittsburgh sleep quality index (PSQI) and selected questions. *Notes* Higher scores reflect worse symptom severity except in the case of sleep duration which is measured in hours. *Significance* $^{**}p < 0.01$. For ratio and quasi-interval scales, means and standard errors are displayed, while medians are displayed for ordinal scales. *Source* Nacasch et al. (2023, p. 5)

no life-threatening events, in line with evidence from similar patient cohorts. Alongside positive changes in PROMs, this suggests CBMPs were well tolerated and adverse events manageable. Moreover, patients with previous exposure to cannabis continue to benefit after initiating treatment with CBMPs. However, owing to limitations discussed in this study, definitive conclusions on efficacy or causality are limited and results should be interpreted considering the subjectivity of PROMs.

2.5 West Syndrome

One study, published by Caraballo and Valenzuela (2021), was identified from the PubMed search that described the potential therapeutic benefits of medical cannabis for children with treatment-resistant West syndrome. Caraballo and Valenzuela retrospectively analysed the medical records of eight children whose West syndrome was untreatable. The medical cannabis treatment that the children received was a ration of cannabidiol: Δ-9-tetrahydrocannabinol (CBD:THC) of 25:1. The length of time for their study was from May 2020 to March 2021. At the beginning of the study, participants received an initial dose of 2 mg/kg/day and this dosage was gradually increased to a maximum of 12 mg/kg/day. They observed that:

> Prior to CBD initiation, patients had a mean of 63 seizures per day (range, 31–79). After a follow-up of between 6 and 13 months, a 75–99% decrease in seizure frequency was observed in two patients, a 50–74% decrease in two, a less than 50% decrease in three, and no changes in seizure frequency were seen in the remaining patient. … Adverse effects were mild and transient. Somnolence was observed in one patient, nausea and vomiting in one, and behavior disturbances and irritability in another patient. (Caraballo & Valenzuela, 2021, p. 238)

2.6 Sleep Disorders/Insomnia

Six studies were identified from the retrieved citations from the PubMed search that contained descriptions about the therapeutic potential of medical cannabis on insomnia and sleep disturbances (AminiLari et al., 2022; Murphy et al., 2023; Ried et al., 2023; Suraev et al., 2023; Sznitman et al., 2022; Walsh et al., 2021). Details about these studies and their results are now outlined.

AminiLari et al. (2022) published a systematic review and meta-analysis of randomised clinical trials about medicinal cannabis and cannabinoids for impaired sleep. They searched for relevant studies that were hosted on MEDLINE, EMBASE, CENTRAL, and PsycINFO. All articles stored on these databases until 19 January 2021 were screened. To be included in their systematic review and meta-analysis, the study had to:

1. be randomised controlled trial,
2. have participants aged 18 years or older with impaired sleep,
3. have the participants randomised to any form of medical cannabis or cannabinoid vs. non-cannabis control, and
4. report data that was collected > 14 days after treatment.

Studies were excluded if they were open-label trails, studies that enrolled participants using cannabis for recreational purposes, and studies in which the participants were taking medical cannabis for cannabis use disorder or cannabis withdrawal (AminiLari et al., 2022). They identified and examined 39 trials, that had a pooled group of 5100 participants. Of these trials, for 38 trials participants consumed oral cannabinoids and for the other trial the participants used inhaled cannabis. Across all trials, 35 days was the median follow-up after discontinuation of cannabis treatment. Within most trials (i.e., 33 of 39), enrolled patients were diagnosed with either chronic cancer or noncancer chronic pain. They discovered that medical cannabis usage helped the participants with these conditions obtain mild improvements in their quality of sleep. They concluded that:

> We found moderate to high certainty evidence that, when compared to placebo, use of medical cannabis or cannabinoids results in small improvements in sleep quality among patients living with chronic pain; small improvements in sleep disturbance among patients living with chronic noncancer pain, very small improvement in sleep disturbance among chronic cancer pain patients, and small increases in several adverse side effects (with a large increase in dizziness with longer treatment). The effects of medical cannabis and cannabinoids on

impaired sleep, compared to active treatment, is uncertain as the evidence is only low to very low certainty. (AminiLari et al., 2022, p. 9)

Murphy et al. (2023) compared the patient-reported outcome measures (PROMs) from patients with impaired sleep who were using cannabis-based medicinal products (CBMPs) for generalised anxiety disorder (GAD) to patients without impaired sleep who were also using CBMPs for GAD. PROMs were collected from participants at the beginning of the study (i.e., baseline) and at one, three, six, and 12 months into the study. Primary outcomes of this study were any clinically significant improvements in GAD scores over the study timeline. Secondary outcomes were any incident and frequency of an adverse event (e.g., chest pain, dizziness, and fatigue). They reported that at all time points the 302 participants that were examined in their study demonstrated an improvement in mean GAD-7, single-item sleep quality, and EQ-5D-5L index scores ($p < 0.001$). They also discovered that 55 (18.21%) participants reported a total of 707 adverse events. They concluded that CBMP treatment contributed to improvements in anxiety among participants diagnosed with GAD. Additionally, although CBMP gave participants with comorbid sleep disruption greater improvements in anxiety, this statistical finding was not sustained when a multivariate analysis was performed. Finally, they concluded that a predictor for CBMP treatment outcomes may be the severity of anxiety at baseline (Murphy et al., 2023).

Ried et al. (2023) conducted a six-week randomised crossover double-blind placebo-controlled trial to determine whether the insomnia experienced by adults can be treated by Entoura-10:15 medicinal cannabis oil. A total of 29 participants who had declared that they had clinical insomnia completed the crossover trial. All participants were randomised to receive either placebo or active oil that contains 10 mg/ml tetrahydrocannabinol (THC) and 15 mg/ml cannabidiol (CBD) over a two-week period. The dosages were titrated from 0.2 to 1.5 m/day, and this was followed by a one-week wash-out period before crossover. The tolerability of THL and CBD was documented by the participants through daily diary entries. Melatonin levels in saliva measured at midnight, data collected from Fitbit activity/sleep wrist trackers, and reliable questionnaires (e.g., *Insomnia Severity Index*) were used to determine the effectiveness of THC and CBD in helping participants manage their insomnia (Ried et al., 2023).

Within the experimental group (i.e., those who received Entoura-10:15 medicinal cannabis oil), melatonin levels at midnight significantly increased by 30% compared to a 20% decline in the placebo group (i.e., those who did not take Entoura-10:15 medicinal cannabis oil) (see Fig. 2.3). They also discovered that at the end of the two-week intervention component of the study 60% of participants in the experimental group were no longer eligible to be diagnosed with clinical insomnia compared to less than 40% in the placebo group (see Fig. 2.4). Within the experimental group, the duration and quality of light sleep increased by an average of 21 min per night compared to the placebo group ($p = 0.041$) (see Fig. 2.5). Thus, they concluded that Entoura-10:15 medicinal cannabis oil was generally well tolerated and effective in improving sleep (Ried et al., 2023).

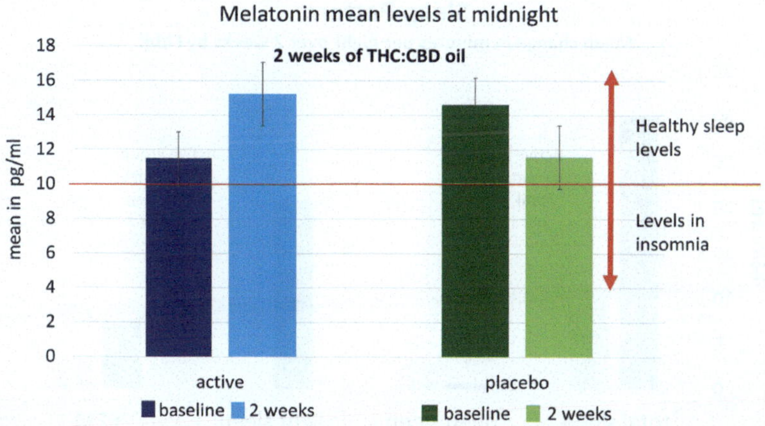

Fig. 2.3 Midnight melatonin levels before and after 2-week intervention. *Notes* Dark blue = active baseline, light blue = active 2 weeks, dark green = placebo baseline, light green = placebo 2 weeks; red line = threshold level, melatonin < 10 pg/ml is considered deficient and associated with insomnia. CBD, cannabidiol; THC, delta-9-tetrahydrocannabinol. *Source* Ried et al. (2023, p. 7)

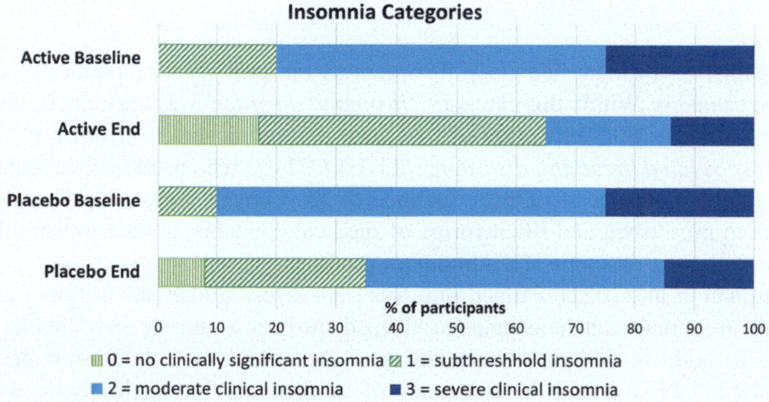

Fig. 2.4 Insomnia categories before and after intervention by group. *Notes* Categories in bar graph: 0 = no clinical insomnia (striped light green), 1 = sub-threshold insomnia (striped dark green), 2 = moderate clinical insomnia (solid light blue), 3 = severe clinical insomnia (solid dark blue). Insomnia categories are based on the Insomnia Severity Index score. We enrolled primarily adults with clinical insomnia (groups 2 and 3). In all, 60% of participants were no longer classified as clinical insomniacs at the end of the trial. *Source* Ried et al. (2023, p. 8)

Suraev et al. (2023) investigated the demographics and traits of a sample of Australians who reported using medically prescribed and/or illicit cannabis to manage their self-identified sleep disorders. To achieve this objective, they performed a subanalysis utilising data from the cross-sections *Cannabis as Medicine Survey 2020–2021*, that involved 1600 participants. Most participants ($n = 1030$ out of 1600

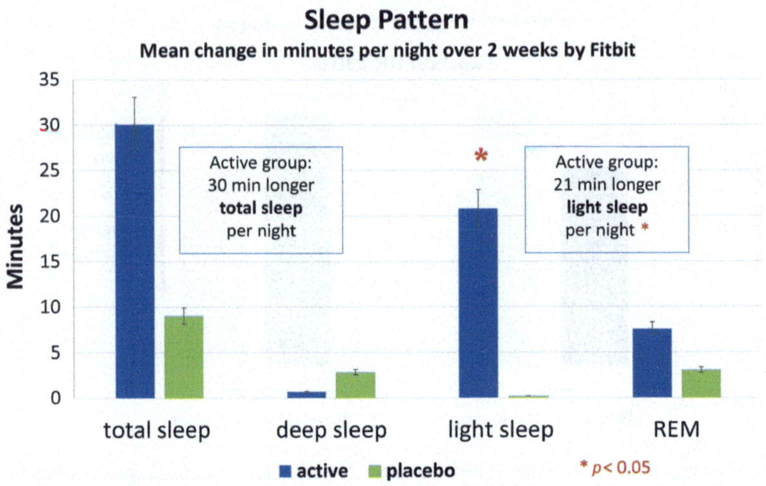

Fig. 2.5 Change in sleep pattern over time. *Notes* Length in min/night and by sleep stage (total, deep, light, rapid eye movement [REM]) assessed by Fitbit wrist activity tracker. Blue bars (active), green bars (placebo). Light sleep significantly improved by 21 min/night in the active group. *Source* Ried et al. (2023, p. 9)

participants, 64%) identified sleep disorders as the primary therapeutic target for medical cannabis. Within this category, '*insomnia disorder*' was the most frequently selected subtype (85.5%), followed by '*sleep-related movement disorders*' (26%) and '*sleep-related breathing disorders*' (11.1%). Those who used medical cannabis to treat sleep disorders were more inclined to be younger, a greater probability of using both prescribed and illicit forms of medical cannabis, tended to use inhaled routes of administration to THC-dominant products.

Sznitman et al. (2022) claimed that there are a few studies about how medical cannabis treatment can help manage sleep disturbances among participants with PTSD. To address this gap, Sznitman et al. examined the relationship between medical cannabis use and the frequency of awakenings during the night, waking up early, and experiencing nightmares. Over a span of two weeks, every morning 77 participants taking medical cannabis to manage their PTSD recorded when they consumed medical cannabis the previous night and any sleep disturbances that they experienced. They discovered that the prospect of experiencing nightmares was reduced if there was a shorter interval between medical cannabis use and the onset of sleep. However, this interval did not decrease the occurrence of nightly awakenings or premature awakening. However, participants using medical cannabis products with greater concentrations of CBD reported fewer instances of early awakenings. They concluded that:

> Our data suggest that MC may help reduce nightmares and CBD in particular may be important for preventing early awakenings. This provides a strong basis for further hypotheses testing, potentially through clinical trials, of the sleep-inducing effects of MC and for testing CBD in particular. Given the high comorbidity of PTSD symptoms and sleep disturbances

> and the potential for MC to have effects on both, a greater understanding of how patients experience the effects of MC on overall PTSD symptoms and sleep disturbances is warranted. (Sznitman et al., 2022, p. 6)

Walsh et al. (2021) evaluated the safety and efficacy of two weeks usage of ZTL-101, a cannabinoid extract in treating chronic insomnia (i.e., as defined as insomnia symptoms $\geq$ 3 months) among 24 participants. They measured adverse events, global insomnia symptoms (i.e., as gauged by the *Insomnia Severity Index*), and a self-reported sleep diary. Wake after sleep onset, total sleep time, sleep efficacy, and sleep onset latency. They reported that no adverse events were identified. However, 40 mild, nonserious, adverse events were identified, of which 36 occurred during ZTL-101 treatment. These events often resolved overnight or soon after waking. Despite these mild concerns, ZTL-101 was found to be an effective treatment in managing chronic insomnia. Similar results were reported by the studies examined by Sarris et al. (2020) (see Appendix C).

2.7 Depression

Two studies about the therapeutic benefits that medical cannabis provided patients with depression were identified from the citations collected from the PubMed search (Mangoo et al., 2022; Sachedina et al., 2022). Mangoo et al. (2022) measured the safety and impact that prescribed cannabis-based medicinal products (CBMPs) had on the health-related quality of life (HRQoL) among patients with depression. Participants were sourced from the UK Medical Cannabis Registry. Changes in scores from baseline to one, three, and six months in *Patient Health Questionnaire-9* (PHQ-9), *Generalised Anxiety Disorder-7* (GAD-7), *Sleep Quality Scale* (SQS), and *EQ-5D-5L* were the primary outcomes measured. The secondary outcomes measured were the occurrence of adverse events. They identified 129 patients from the UK Medical Cannabis Registry. They discovered that there was an improvement in PHQ-9, GAD-7, SQS, and EQ-5D-5L scores. They also identified 153 adverse events ($n = 133$ out of 153, 87%) classified as *'moderate'* to *'mild'*. Similar results were reported by the studies examined by Sarris et al. (2020) (see Appendix C).

Sachedina et al. (2022) examined the impact that medical cannabis had on the anxiety and depression symptoms of 7,362 participants (average age = 49.8 years; 53.1% female). All participants completed the GAD-7 and PHQ-9 at the initial evaluation and at one point during the follow-up visit. From baseline to follow-up, both GAD-7 and PHQ-9 scores improved. Due to the size of the sample, it is plausible to argue that the generalisability of the results can be applied to the broader population.

2.8 Treatment-Resistant Epilepsy

One study, published by Erridge et al. (2023), was retrieved from the PubMed search that documented the efficacy of cannabis-based medicinal products (CBMPs) to manage treatment-resistant epilepsy among children. The results of their study were based on 35 patients who were on the UK Medical Cannabis Registry. The primary outcome that they measured was a $\geq$ 50% reduction in seizure frequency, changes in the *Impact of Paediatric Epilepsy Score*, and the occurrence of adverse events. Overall, 23 (65.7%) participants achieved $a \geq 50\%$ reduction in seizure frequency. They also discovered that most patients (n = 16 out of 17, 94.1%) treated with CBD and Δ^9-THC combination therapy experienced $a \geq 50\%$ reduction in the frequency of seizures. In comparison, 31.6% (n = 6 out of 19) participants treated with CBD isolates and 17.6% (n = 3 out of 17) participants treated with broader-spectrum CBD products experienced a $\geq$ 50% reduction in the frequency of seizures. Additionally, most adverse events were classified as '*mild*' (n = 12), followed by '*moderate*' (n = 10), '*severe*' (n = 3), and '*debilitating or life threatening*' (n = 1) (see Table 2.1).

Table 2.1 Adverse events reported by participants (n = 39)

Adverse events	Mild	Moderate	Severe	Debilitating/life threatening	Total
Anorexia	0	0	1	0	1 (2.9%)
Anxiety	0	1	0	0	1 (2.9%)
Constipation	1	0	0	0	1 (2.9%)
Fatigue	11	3	0	0	14 (40.0%)
Lethargy	0	1	0	0	1 (2.9%)
Nausea	0	0	1	0	1 (2.9%)
Seizure frequency increased	0	2	0	0	2 (5.7%)
Sepsis	0	0	0	1	1 (2.9%)
Somnolence	0	2	0	0	2 (5.7%)
Vomiting	0	1	0	0	1 (2.9%)
Weight loss	0	0	1	0	1 (2.9%)
Total	12 (34.2%)	10 (28.6%)	3 (8.6%)	1 (2.9%)	26 (74.3%)

Source Erridge et al. (2023, p. 178)

2.9 Brain Injury

Hergert et al. (2021) published a review of the literature about high-quality studies that contained descriptions about the benefits and adverse events that people with traumatic brain injury (TBI) encounter after using medical cannabis. They discovered that the studies that they examined described a diverse range of benefits. For example, Hawley et al. (2018) reported that among participants with TBI 62% who used cannabis reported a reduction in anxiety and 55% reported improved sleep. Additionally, McVige et al. (2019) reported that medical cannabis was associated with improved quality of sleep and quality of life, reduced headache occurrences, and a decrease among patients with a history of concussion using opioid medications. Based on these eclectic findings, Hergert et al. (2021, p. 1913) concluded that:

> In conclusion, medical cannabis may represent a viable treatment for TBI, but the research is very much in its infancy. The lack of high-quality experimental studies makes it difficult to draw concrete conclusions about the positive and negative effects of medical cannabis on TBI. Pre-clinical studies of medical cannabis demonstrating its neuroprotective qualities have yet to translate into human studies, mainly because very few studies on the topic exist. This review has identified several key research directions in TBI in the topics of neuroimaging, cognition, psychiatric, and physical symptoms that need to be addressed.

2.10 Autism Spectrum Disorders

Four studies were identified from the PubMed search that contained descriptions about the therapeutic benefits and adverse events that medical cannabis gives autistic people (Ben-Zeev, 2020; Efron & Taylor, 2023; Erridge et al., 2022; Fletcher et al., 2022; Holdman et al., 2022). What follows now is a description of these studies and a presentation of their results.

Efron and Taylor (2023) reviewed the literature about the benefits and drawbacks that medical cannabis had on people with developmental, behavioural, and mental health disorders. They searched for clinical trials on Australian and New Zealand Trial Registry, clinicaltrials.gov, ISRCTN, and the EU Clinical Trials Register. They excluded single-case studies and conference abstracts. They identified seven studies about the clinical benefits and drawbacks that medicinal cannabis gave autistics. Despite these mixed results, they concluded that:

> Adverse events are largely described as mild; most commonly, they are appetite changes, somnolence, or worsened behavioural or anxiety symptoms. Only one study reported a serious adverse event, psychosis, considered to be related to the higher THC content given to that participant. Although these preliminary reports are promising, several of these studies are limited by small sample sizes or insufficient follow-up of participants who discontinued treatment, and all are limited by being open-label or observational studies. Double-blind placebo-controlled trials are needed to test efficacy scientifically. (Efron & Taylor, 2023, p. 2)

Erridge et al. (2022) published a case series that described changes to HRQoL and the incidence of adverse events while using CBMPs among autistic patients on the UK Medical Cannabis Registry. Participants completed the GAD-7, SQS, and EQ-5D-5L at baseline and at one, three, and six months into the study. Adverse events were also recorded and analysed. Data was collected from 74 autistic participants. HRQoL and sleep improved at one and three months, as indicated by EQ-5D-5L, SQS, and GAD-7. Improvements in HRQoL and sleep were sustained at six months into the study, as indicated by the SQS and EQ-5D-5L. Out of the 74 participants in their study, 14 (18.9%) participants reported a total of 180 adverse events. Most adverse events were classified as '*moderate*' ($n = 81$), followed by '*mild*' ($n = 58$) and '*severe*' ($n = 41$). The most common adverse event reported was '*insomnia*' ($n = 13$) (see Table 2.2). Based on these results, they concluded that:

> In this first published experience of clinical outcomes in adult patients with ASD treated with CBMPs, there were associated improvements in general health-related quality of life, in addition to sleep- and anxiety-specific outcomes. Moreover, there was a reduction in the administration of concomitant medications, some of which are associated with serious adverse events with long-term use. CBMPs were well tolerated by the majority (81.1%) of patients. (Erridge et al., 2022, p. 9)

Fletcher et al. (2022) conducted a scoping review to identify and report the results in the literature about the benefits and adverse events of autistics using medicinal cannabis. They identified eight completed and five ongoing studies. They discovered that autistics who consumed medicinal cannabis experienced improvements with anxiety, communication, hyperactivity, behavioural changes, seizures, and sleep. Despite these benefits, Fletcher et al. discovered that within the studies that they examined autistics reported adverse events, including confusion and tremors.

Holdman et al. (2022) compared the safety and efficacy of medications commonly used to assist autistics to that of medical cannabis. They discovered that the heterogeneity of the symptoms associated with the autism spectrum undermines the ability to find any suitable treatment. Such difficulty results in patients trying many medication changes and treatment trials. They also discovered that the US Food and Drug Administration has only approved two medications to help autistics manage their irritability. Finally, they discovered that there were no published placebo-controlled trial of autistics using medical cannabis, which undermines the ability to create any robust conclusions as to the long-term safety of medical cannabis for autistics. Despite this finding, preliminary research indicates that CBD-rich medical cannabis appears to be an effective, tolerable, and relative safety. It also appears to help autistics manage irritability and sleeping problems.

2.11 Multiple Sclerosis

One study was identified from the PubMed search in which the therapeutic potential of medical cannabis for patients with multiple sclerosis (Rainka et al., 2023). Rainka et al. (2023) conducted a retrospective medical record review of 141 people with multiple sclerosis who were receiving medications to manage their symptoms of multiple sclerosis. After medical cannabis treatment started, data was collected at

Table 2.2 Adverse events reported by participants

Adverse event	Mild	Moderate	Severe	Total
Abdominal pain (upper)	1	1	1	3 (4.1%)
Agitation	–	1	2	3 (4.1%)
Amnesia	1	3	1	5 (6.8%)
Anorexia	–	3	3	6 (8.1%)
Anxiety	–	–	1	1 (1.4%)
Ataxia	3	1	1	5 (6.8%)
Blurred vision	1	3	2	6 (8.1%)
Cognitive disturbance	1	2	2	5 (6.8%)
Concentration impairment	5	4	1	10 (13.5%)
Confusion	–	–	2	2 (2.7%)
Constipation	–	1	–	1 (1.4%)
Delirium	1	–	1	2 (2.7%)
Depression	–	–	4	4 (5.4%)
Diarrhoea	–	1	–	1 (1.4%)
Dizziness	2	2	1	5 (6.8%)
Dry mouth	10	1	–	11 (14.9%)
Dysgeusia	1	1	2	4 (5.4%)
Dyspepsia	4	2	–	6 (8.1%)
Fall	–	2	–	2 (2.7%)
Fatigue	3	3	4	10 (13.5%)
Fasciculations	–	1	–	1 (1.4%)
Generalised muscle weakness	2	2	1	5 (6.8%)
Headache	–	7	1	8 (10.8%)
Increased seizure frequency	–	1	2	3 (4.1%)
Insomnia	2	7	4	13 (17.6%)
Lethargy	3	7	1	11 (14.9%)
Nausea	4	2	–	6 (8.1%)
Pharyngitis	–	3	–	3 (4.1%)
Pyrexia	–	1	–	1 (1.4%)
Rash	2	–	–	2 (2.7%)
Somnolence	–	9	–	9 (12.2%)
Spasticity	2	3	1	6 (8.1%)
Tremor	5	–	2	7 (9.5%)
Vertigo	2	1	1	4 (5.4%)
Vomiting	2	–	–	2 (2.7%)
Weight loss	1	3	–	4 (5.4%)

(continued)

Table 2.2 (continued)

Adverse event	Mild	Moderate	Severe	Total
Upper respiratory tract infection	–	3	–	3 (4.1%)
Total	58 (78.4%)	81 (109.5%)	41 (55.4%)	180 (243.2%)

Source Erridge et al. (2022, pp. 7–8)

four follow-up appointments. Indicators of the effectiveness of medical cannabis were medication changes, changes in cognition and mobility, symptoms of multiple sclerosis, and adverse events. They discovered that after being on medical cannabis treatment patients reported reductions in pain (72% of patients), spasticity (48% of patients), and sleep problems (40% of patients). However, they also discovered that the most adverse side effects of medical cannabis treatment were fatigue (11% of patients). Based on these results, they concluded that:

> This study shows that MC may help decrease chronic pain, muscle spasticity, and sleep disturbances in patients with MS, and patients may also be able to reduce opioid use during MC treatment. Users of MC may require individualized therapy to balance efficacy and AEs. Prospective studies of the effects of MC on MS symptoms and opioid use would be beneficial, and, ultimately, could influence future legislation as it pertains to the legalization of MC in the United States. (Rainka et al., 2023, p. 116)

2.12 Parkinson's Disease

Bougea et al.'s (2020) study was the only study identified from the PubMed search that described the therapeutic effectiveness of medical cannabis for people with Parkinson's disease. Bougea et al. conducted a systematic review of the literature with the intention of evaluating the efficacy of medical cannabis for people with Parkinson's disease and evaluating the quality of research collected. They evaluated the findings and quality of 14 studies. They discovered that five studies reported that medical cannabis had positive therapeutic benefits on the motor abilities of people with Parkinson's disease and four studies reported positive benefits on non-motor symptoms. They concluded that:

> Despite the increasing use of cannabis for PD, there is a lack of consensus regarding the efficacy and scope of adverse effects of the drug, and this is reflected in the diverse recommendations for its use across different countries. Collectively, current data suggest that there is insufficient evidence to recommend the use of cannabis for the motor symptoms in PD, while its safety still remains unclear. Currently, until further controlled studies are performed, and until the long-term results are known, the use of MC should not be encouraged, except in the context of an investigational trial or in very select patients with refractory non-motor symptoms, such as pain. There is a need for well designed RTCs of cannabis with a larger sample to establish evidence based data, which will inform MC legislation. (Bougea et al., 2020, p. 8).

2.13 Gilles De La Tourette

One study was identified from the PubMed search that contained descriptions about the therapeutic benefits that medical cannabis gave people with Gilles de la Tourette syndrome (Anis et al., 2022). Anis et al. (2022) examined the benefits and tolerability of medical cannabis treatment for Gilles de la Tourette syndrome. Their study was an open-label, prospective study, and the use of medical cannabis was determined by the participant's treating neurologist. At the beginning of the study, each participant completed the *Yale Global Tic Severity Scale* (YGTSS) and the baseline score was 60.3 ± 17.1 (range 0–100). At 4 and 12 weeks after the participants began medical cannabis treatment, the efficacy, tolerability, and side effects of medical cannabis were assessed. At the beginning of the study, 18 participants were enrolled. However, three participants did not complete the study. Smoking cannabis was the most common way that medical cannabis was consumed (80%). They discovered that after 12 weeks of medical cannabis treatment there was a 38% average reduction in YGTSS scores. They also discovered that there was a 20% reduction in the *Premonitory Urge for Tic Scale*. Dry mouth (66.7%), fatigue (53.3%), and dizziness (46.7%) were the most common side effects reported by the participants (see Fig. 2.6). Worsening of obsessive–compulsive disorder (which resulted in the participant stopping treatment), panic attacks, and anxiety (which the participant took medications to treat) were common psychiatric side effects reported by three participants. Additionally, cognitive side effects of distorted time perception, visuospatial disorientation, confusion, slow processing speed, and attention were reported by six participants. Finally, improvements were observed on the subjective effectiveness of medical cannabis on tics and quality of life (see Fig. 2.7) (Anis et al., 2022). Based on these results, Anis et al. (2022, p. 8) concluded that:

> Our results are in line with a number of other studies suggesting that MC is effective and well tolerated in adults with GTS. From our data, it is suggested that MC might be a treatment option for resistant TS patients, and MC has a significant effect on tics, premonitory urges, and patients' overall quality of life. In our sample, patients favored THC-rich cannabis strands and smoking/inhaling MC over sublingual oil. One has to be aware of the neurological and cognitive SEs of MC and monitor them during treatment. The limitations of our study due to the open, uncontrolled design emphasize the necessity for controlled studies to further evaluate the role of MC in this disorder.

2.14 Conclusion

This chapter presented a summary of the literature about the therapeutic benefits and drawbacks of using medical/medicinal cannabis. It was discovered that under certain circumstances medical/medicinal cannabis has the potential to improve the quality of life for people with various disabilities and psychiatric and medical conditions. For example, it was discovered that it can help people with Gilles de la Tourette manage the frequency of their tics. Despite these potential benefits, it should be noted that

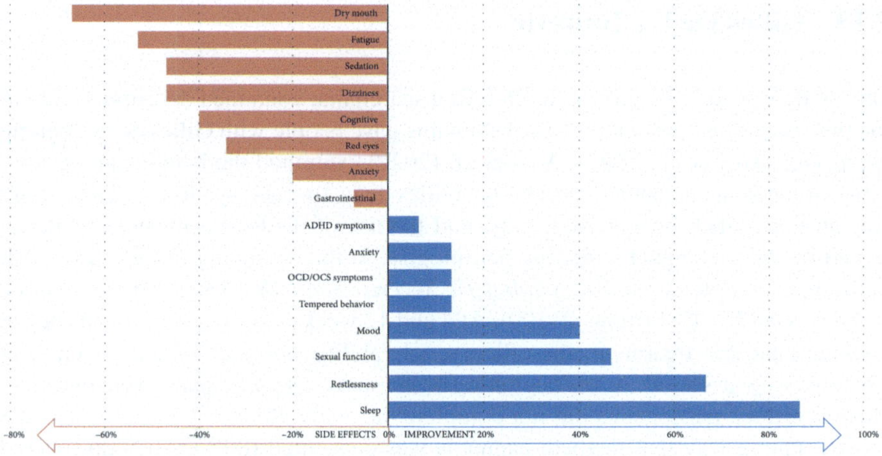

Fig. 2.6 Treatment-related side effects and influence on comorbidities and life habits. *OCS* obsessive compulsive symptoms; *OCD* obsessive compulsive disorder; *ADHD* attention-deficit hyperactive disorder. *Source* Anis et al. (2022, p. 8)

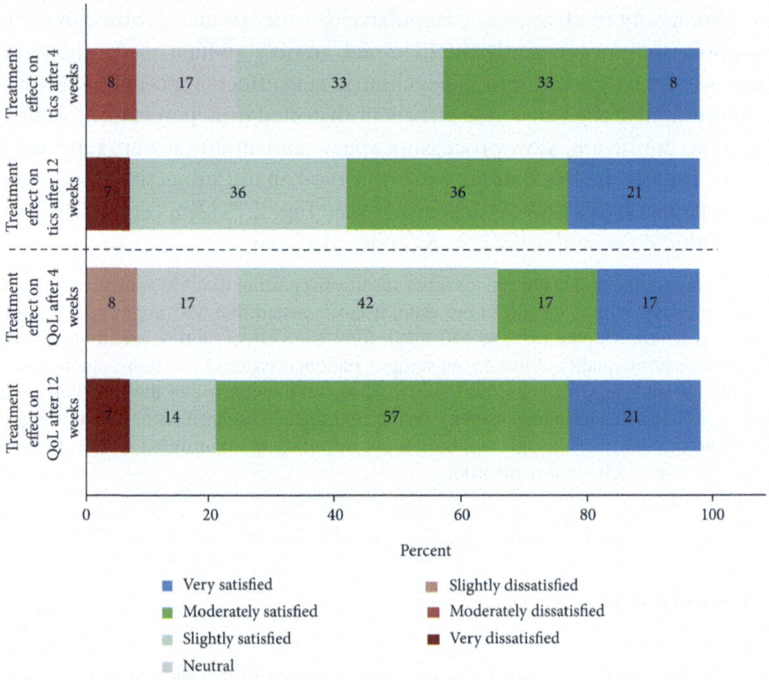

Fig. 2.7 Subjective effectiveness of MC on tics and QoL using a 7-point Likert-type scale. *MC* medical cannabis; *QoL* quality of life. *Source* Anis et al. (2022, p. 6)

only a few studies were identified for each disability and psychiatric or medical condition. Thus, for these results to be validated it is prudent that more research is conducted.

References

AminiLari, M., Wang, L., Neumark, S., Adli, T., Couban, R. J., Giangregorio, A., Carney, C. E., & Busse, J. W. (2022). Medical cannabis and cannabinoids for impaired sleep: A systematic review and meta-analysis of randomized clinical trials. *Sleep, 45*(2), zsab234. https://doi.org/10.1093/sleep/zsab234

Anis, S., Zalomek, C., Korczyn, A. D., Rosenberg, A., Giladi, N., & Gurevich, T. (2022). Medical cannabis for Gilles de la Tourette syndrome: An open-label prospective study. *Behavioural Neurology, 2022*, 5141773. https://doi.org/10.1155/2022/5141773

Bapir, L., Erridge, S., Nicholas, M., Pillai, M., Dalavaye, N., Holvey, C., Coomber, R., Hoare, J., Khan, S., Weatherall, M. W., Rucker, J. J., Platt, M., & Sodergren, M. H. (2023). Comparing the effects of medical cannabis for chronic pain patients with and without co-morbid anxiety: A cohort study. *Expert Review of Neurotherapeutics, 23*(3), 281–295. https://doi.org/10.1080/14737175.2023.2181696

Ben-Zeev, B. (2020). Medical cannabis for intractable epilepsy in childhood: A review. *Rambam Maimonides Medical Journal, 11*(1), e0004. https://doi.org/10.5041/RMMJ.10387

Bougea, A., Koros, C., Simitsi, A. M., Chrysovitsanou, C., Leonardos, A., & Stefanis, L. (2020). Medical cannabis as an alternative therapeutics for Parkinsons' disease: Systematic review. *Complementary Therapies in Clinical Practice, 39*, 101154. https://doi.org/10.1016/j.ctcp.2020.101154

Caraballo, R., & Valenzuela, G. R. (2021). Cannabidiol-enriched medical cannabis as add-on therapy in children with treatment-resistant West syndrome: A study of eight patients. *Seizure, 92*, 238–243. https://doi.org/10.1016/j.seizure.2021.10.002

Efron, D., & Taylor, K. (2023). Medicinal cannabis for paediatric developmental, behavioural and mental health disorders. *International Journal of Environmental Research and Public Health, 20*(8), 5430. https://doi.org/10.3390/ijerph20085430

Ergisi, M., Erridge, S., Harris, M., Kawka, M., Nimalan, D., Salazar, O., Loupasaki, K., Ali, R., Holvey, C., Coomber, R., Platt, M., Rucker, J. J., & Sodergren, M. H. (2022). UK Medical cannabis registry: An analysis of clinical outcomes of medicinal cannabis therapy for generalized anxiety disorder. *Expert Review of Clinical Pharmacology, 15*(4), 487–495. https://doi.org/10.1080/17512433.2022.2020640

Erridge, S., Holvey, C., Coomber, R., Hoare, J., Khan, S., Platt, M. W., Rucker, J. J., Weatherall, M. W., Beri, S., & Sodergren, M. H. (2023). Clinical outcome data of children treated with cannabis-based medicinal products for treatment resistant Epilepsy-analysis from the UK medical cannabis registry. *Neuropediatrics, 54*(3), 174–181. https://doi.org/10.1055/a-2002-2119

Erridge, S., Kerr-Gaffney, J., Holvey, C., Coomber, R., Barros, D. A. R., Bhoskar, U., Mwimba, G., Praveen, K., Symeon, C., Sachdeva-Mohan, S., Sodergren, M. H., & Rucker, J. J. (2022). Clinical outcome analysis of patients with autism spectrum disorder: Analysis from the UK medical cannabis registry. *Therapeutic Advances in Psychopharmacology, 12*, 20451253221116240. https://doi.org/10.1177/20451253221116240

Fletcher, S., Pawliuk, C., Ip, A., Huh, L., Rassekh, S. R., Oberlander, T. F., & Siden, H. (2022). Medicinal cannabis in children and adolescents with autism spectrum disorder: A scoping review. *Child: Care, Health and Development*, *48*(1), 33–44. https://doi.org/10.1111/cch.12909

Hawley, L. A., Ketchum, J. M., Morey, C., Collins, K., & Charlifue, S. (2018). Cannabis use in individuals with spinal cord injury or moderate to severe traumatic brain injury in Colorado.

Archives of Physical Medicine and Rehabilitation, 99(8), 1584–1590. https://doi.org/10.1016/j.apmr.2018.02.003

Hergert, D. C., Robertson-Benta, C., Sicard, V., Schwotzer, D., Hutchison, K., Covey, D. P., Quinn, D. K., Sadek, J. R., McDonald, J., & Mayer, A. R. (2021). Use of medical cannabis to treat traumatic brain injury. *Journal of Neurotrauma, 38*(14), 1904–1917. https://doi.org/10.1089/neu.2020.7148

Holdman, R., Vigil, D., Robinson, K., Shah, P., & Contreras, A. E. (2022). Safety and efficacy of medical cannabis in autism spectrum disorder compared with commonly used medications. *Cannabis and Cannabinoid Research, 7*(4), 451–463. https://doi.org/10.1089/can.2020.0154

Ittiphakorn, P., Erridge, S., Holvey, C., Coomber, R., Rucker, J. J., & Sodergren, M. H. (2023). UK medical cannabis registry: An analysis of clinical outcomes of medicinal cannabis therapy for attention-deficit/hyperactivity disorder. *Neuropsychopharmacology Reports, 43*(4), 596–606. https://doi.org/10.1002/npr2.12400

Korb, L., Tromans, S., Perera, B., Khan, N., Burrows, L., Laugharne, R., Hassiotis, A., Allgar, V., Efron, D., Maidment, I., & Shankar, R. (2023). The potential for medicinal cannabis to help manage challenging behaviour in people with intellectual disability: A perspective review. *Journal of Psychopharmacology (Oxford, England), 37*(12), 1201–1208. https://doi.org/10.1177/02698811231209192

Krediet, E., Janssen, D. G., Heerdink, E. R., Egberts, T. C., & Vermetten, E. (2020). Experiences with medical cannabis in the treatment of veterans with PTSD: Results from a focus group discussion. *European Neuropsychopharmacology: The Journal of the European College of Neuropsychopharmacology, 36*, 244–254. https://doi.org/10.1016/j.euroneuro.2020.04.009

Mangoo, S., Erridge, S., Holvey, C., Coomber, R., Barros, D. A. R., Bhoskar, U., Mwimba, G., Praveen, K., Symeon, C., Sachdeva-Mohan, S., Rucker, J. J., & Sodergren, M. H. (2022). Assessment of clinical outcomes of medicinal cannabis therapy for depression: Analysis from the UK medical cannabis registry. *Expert Review of Neurotherapeutics, 22*(11–12), 995–1008. https://doi.org/10.1080/14737175.2022.2161894

McVige, J., Kaur, D., Hart, P., Lillis, M., Mechtler, L., Bargnes, V., & Shukri, S. (2019). Medical cannabis in the treatment of post-traumatic concussion (P3. 9-027). *Neurology, 92*(15_supplement), 3–9.

Murphy, M., Erridge, S., Holvey, C., Coomber, R., Rucker, J. J., & Sodergren, M. H. (2023). A cohort study comparing the effects of medical cannabis for anxiety patients with and without comorbid sleep disturbance. *Neuropsychopharmacology Reports*. https://doi.org/10.1002/npr2.12407

Nacasch, N., Avni, C., & Toren, P. (2023). Medical cannabis for treatment-resistant combat PTSD. *Frontiers in Psychiatry, 13*, 1014630. https://doi.org/10.3389/fpsyt.2022.1014630

Pillai, M., Erridge, S., Bapir, L., Nicholas, M., Dalavaye, N., Holvey, C., Coomber, R., Barros, D., Bhoskar, U., Mwimba, G., Praveen, K., Symeon, C., Sachdeva-Mohan, S., Rucker, J. J., & Sodergren, M. H. (2022). Assessment of clinical outcomes in patients with post-traumatic stress disorder: Analysis from the UK medical cannabis registry. *Expert Review of Neurotherapeutics, 22*(11–12), 1009–1018. https://doi.org/10.1080/14737175.2022.2155139

Rainka, M. M., Aladeen, T. S., Mattle, A. G., Lewandowski, E., Vanini, D., McCormack, K., & Mechtler, L. (2023). Multiple sclerosis and use of medical cannabis: A retrospective review of a neurology outpatient population. *International Journal of MS Care, 25*(3), 111–117. https://doi.org/10.7224/1537-2073.2022-006

Ried, K., Tamanna, T., Matthews, S., & Sali, A. (2023). Medicinal cannabis improves sleep in adults with insomnia: A randomised double-blind placebo-controlled crossover study. *Journal of Sleep Research, 32*(3), e13793. https://doi.org/10.1111/jsr.13793

Rifkin-Zybutz, R., Erridge, S., Holvey, C., Coomber, R., Gaffney, J., Lawn, W., Barros, D., Bhoskar, U., Mwimba, G., Praveen, K., Symeon, C., Sachdeva-Mohan, S., Rucker, J. J., & Sodergren, M. H. (2023). Clinical outcome data of anxiety patients treated with cannabis-based medicinal products in the United Kingdom: A cohort study from the UK medical cannabis registry. *Psychopharmacology (Berl), 240*(8), 1735–1745. https://doi.org/10.1007/s00213-023-06399-3

Sachedina, F., Chan, C., Damji, R. S., & de Sanctis, O. J. (2022). Medical cannabis use in Canada and its impact on anxiety and depression: A retrospective study. *Psychiatry Research, 313*, 114573. https://doi.org/10.1016/j.psychres.2022.114573

Sarris, J., Sinclair, J., Karamacoska, D., Davidson, M., & Firth, J. (2020). Medicinal cannabis for psychiatric disorders: A clinically-focused systematic review. *BMC Psychiatry, 20*(1), 24. https://doi.org/10.1186/s12888-019-2409-8

Suraev, A., Mills, L., Abelev, S. V., Arkell, T. R., Lintzeris, N., & McGregor, I. S. (2023). Medical cannabis use patterns for sleep disorders in Australia: Results of the cross-sectional CAMS-20 survey. *Nature and Science of Sleep, 15*, 245–255. https://doi.org/10.2147/NSS.S390583

Sznitman, S. R., Meiri, D., Amit, B. H., Rosenberg, D., & Greene, T. (2022). Posttraumatic stress disorder, sleep and medical cannabis treatment: A daily diary study. *Journal of Anxiety Disorders, 92*, 102632. https://doi.org/10.1016/j.janxdis.2022.102632

Walsh, J. H., Maddison, K. J., Rankin, T., Murray, K., McArdle, N., Ree, M. J., Hillman, D. R., & Eastwood, P. R. (2021). Treating insomnia symptoms with medicinal cannabis: A randomized, crossover trial of the efficacy of a cannabinoid medicine compared with placebo. *Sleep, 44*(11), zsab149. https://doi.org/10.1093/sleep/zsab149

Chapter 3
Views Among Healthcare Professionals and Patients About Medical Cannabis

Abstract This chapter presents the experiences, beliefs, and insights of various healthcare professionals about prescribing medical/medicinal cannabis to their patients. The healthcare professionals canvassed in this chapter are general practitioners, physicians, pharmacists, and psychiatrists. This chapter concludes with a presentation of the results in the literature about the views, beliefs, and experiences of patients using medical/medicinal cannabis.

Keywords Healthcare professionals · Medical cannabis · Medical cannabis policies · Narrative of medical cannabis · Patients · Physicians' perceptions

3.1 General Practitioners and Physicians

Of the 683 citations obtained from the PubMed search, 15 publications contained descriptions of the experiences and/or views of general practitioners or physicians about prescribing medical/medicinal cannabis (Adler et al., 2022; Alharbi et al., 2023; Bawa et al., 2022; Bui et al., 2023; Cheng et al., 2022; Dassieu et al., 2023; Gunning et al., 2022; Hallinan et al., 2021; Hordowicz et al., 2021; Manoharan et al., 2022; Mansell et al., 2022; Ng et al., 2021, 2022; Rønne et al., 2021; Rosenbaek et al., 2023). What follows now is a description of these studies and their results.

Adler et al. (2022) examined the attitudes and knowledge primary care physicians (PCPs) in Israel regarding medical cannabis and their attitudes towards prescribing it for different medical conditions. Alder et al. distributed a survey to PCPs in Israel and 201 completed and returned the survey. They discovered that 51% of respondents believed that medical cannabis was an effective treatment, 63% revealed that they had a scant amount of knowledge about medical cannabis, and 75% expressed the view that they would like to learn more about medical cannabis. Most respondents (61%) were willing to prescribe medical cannabis to dying patients, and fewer than half of all respondents were willing to prescribe medical cannabis for various other conditions. Based on these results, Alder et al. (2022, p. 63) concluded that:

G. Bennett, *A Scoping Review of Clinical Studies About the Therapeutic Benefits of Medical Cannabis*, https://doi.org/10.1007/978-981-97-7941-3_3

In this study we examined PCPs' attitudes and knowledge regarding MC. PCPs in our survey had mixed opinions about its effectiveness and safety profile. The wide range of opinions in this study indicates that the debate about MC is far from being solved. Lack of knowledge emerged as a widespread phenomenon. PCPs were willing to initiate MC treatment for dying patients only; however, renewal of prescriptions was more acceptable. Currently, PCPs in Israel are not authorized to prescribe MC to their patients. If a change in health policy is considered, education programs for improving knowledge should be provided as well as addressing physicians' concerns regarding their personal safety.

From February 2020 to February 2021, Alharbi et al. (2023) surveyed 249 physicians who worked at King Abdulaziz Medical City, Saudi Arabia, about their knowledge of medical cannabis. They examined their perceptions of the therapeutic effects of medical cannabis, their beliefs about its potential harm, and their willingness to prescribe if it was to be legal in future. They discovered that 21% ($n = 64$) felt comfortable prescribing medical cannabis to their patients while 32% ($n = 100$) were indifferent, and 47% ($n = 146$) were not willing to prescribe medical cannabis to their patients. Additionally, most respondents (55%, $n = 170$) were unaware of the different medicinal cannabis products and formulations currently available. In contrast, 23% ($n = 72$) were aware of this information. Based on these and other results, Alharbi et al. (2023, p. 543) concluded that:

the majority of the sample had a knowledge deficit about the medicinal use of cannabis for specific indications, its effects, and the different products and formulations currently available. The low level of knowledge highlights the lack of continuing medical education opportunities about MC for healthcare personnel in Saudi Arabia. Inadequate knowledge and discomfort when discussing MC with patients are barriers in the provision of quality patient care services. We recommend the provision of adequate clinical training, guidelines for treatment protocols, and the availability of best clinical practices for the physicians. (Alharbi et al., 2023)

Bui et al. (2023) interviewed 24 physicians who were authorised to prescribe medical cannabis in Pennsylvania. The primary objective of their study was to gauge how prepared these physicians were to prescribe medical cannabis and advise their patients about medical cannabis. They discovered that the physicians that they interviewed were primarily satisfied with the certification process required to prescribe medical cannabis. However, these physicians noted that communication barriers between physicians and confusion about insurance costs. They concluded that physicians needed additional training about the Pennsylvania medical cannabis programme.

Cheng et al. (2022) conducted a systematic search and narrative review to examine studies about healthcare professionals' perspectives on the use of medicinal cannabis to manage chronic pain. They searched for studies within six databases (i.e., MEDLINE, EMBASE, CINAHL, Scopus, Web of Science, and PubMed) from 2001 to 26 March 2021. They identified 26 studies that met their inclusion criteria (see Appendix F). Based on their review of the literature Cheng et al. (2022, p. 730) concluded:

Healthcare professionals appear to rely on their clinical experiences of caring for people living with chronic pain to make decisions about MC use. Healthcare professionals require

> education and training, and clinical guidelines that provide evidence-based information about efficacy and safety, and guidance related to dosage of MC products for chronic pain. Until these gaps are addressed, healthcare professionals are limited in making informed treatment recommendations about MC, may deny a potentially beneficial intervention, divert patients to inappropriate or unnecessary care, and may be unintentionally devaluing the lived experience and preferences of people with chronic pain.

During November and December 2020, Gunning et al. (2022) performed semi-structured interviews to explore the views of physicians practising in Canada about prescribing medical cannabis. An analysis of the interview transcripts showed that physicians recalled recounting authorisation burdens when prescribing medical cannabis, undertaking a risk–benefit calculus before prescribing medical cannabis, the need to conduct more research about medical cannabis, and the importance of clear communication with patients.

Hallinan et al. (2021) explored the perspectives of 21 physicians in Australia about prescribing cannabinoids to patients. The physicians worked in a diverse range of medical fields, including neurology, rheumatology, oncology, pain medicine, psychiatry, public health, and general practice. The participants in their study noted that appropriate regulation, the use of data to evaluate safety and efficacy of medical cannabis, improved prescriber education, and a continuous monitoring of the quality and cost of medical cannabis were important factors to consider.

Hordowicz et al. (2021) explored the knowledge and perspectives of physicians in Poland about medical cannabis. Between June and October 2023, 173 physicians completed their survey. Most participants disclosed that they had never received any education about prescribing medical cannabis (60.1%), that they had limited knowledge to advise their patients about medical cannabis (71.1%), that they would like the knowledge to answer their patients' questions about medical cannabis (92.4%), and that clear guidelines about medical cannabis in clinical practice are needed (93.1%). Based on these and other results Hordowicz et al. (2021, pp. 12–13) concluded that:

> This study is the first insight into the perspectives of Polish physicians regarding the medical applications of cannabinoids. Most medical professionals have expressed their support for the medical use of cannabis and cannabinoids. However, the majority do not feel prepared for patient counseling, which is concerning. They could benefit from targeted educational interventions. Such interventions might encompass independent courses for licensed physicians, congresses, and websites. Additionally, this study has also identified physicians' preferences and suggestions for stakeholders responsible for shaping the policy regarding cannabis-based therapeutics. Further research is encouraged to investigate opinions and knowledge of the representatives of other medical professions (such as pharmacists, nurses, among others); to detect differences among representatives of different medical specialties, such as general practitioners, oncology, and pain specialists; and to identify factors contributing to their choices.

Manoharan et al. (2022) examined the existing beliefs, knowledge, possible concerns, and personal perceptions of medical cannabis among 14 physicians in New Zealand. They discovered that making prescription decisions was predominantly influenced by the physician–patient relationship. Additionally, concerns about possible side effects, the standardisation and quality of medication, and concerns about equitable access to medical cannabis between higher and lower socio-economic patients were the main barriers to prescribing medical cannabis. Finally, some physicians were worried about their liability and risks to their reputation in medical cannabis issues arose for patients. They concluded that:

> The way physicians regard prescribing medical cannabis is based on their personal beliefs and knowledge built up over their medical career. It is important that these are taken into consideration in the design of future guidelines to help alleviate uncertainties and reduce barriers for informed prescribing. While our research and previous research find that physicians generally will follow clinical guidelines based on institutional logics (i.e. the standardised approach to medicine), we find that physicians often allow their personal construals to determine their perceptions and prescribing behaviour to a considerable extent when they practice medicine.

Mansell et al. (2022) conducted a qualitative study to explore the experiences of clinicians who have prescribed medical cannabis to children. Across seven provinces in Canada, 13 physicians were interviewed. Most often children with autism or refractory seizure disorders were prescribed medical cannabis. For example, lack of knowledge about medical cannabis among physicians, stigma associated with taking medical cannabis, and a lack of policies about taking medical cannabis. In contrast, a series of potential solutions were discovered, for example, improving communication with patients about medical cannabis and improving family support about medical cannabis.

Ng et al. (2021) explored the attitudes of family physicians practising in Ontario towards medical cannabis. Between January and October 2019, 11 physicians participated in semi-structured telephone interviews. A thematic analysis of the interview transcripts revealed three main themes, which were: (1) reluctance to authorise medical cannabis, (2) harms associated with the use of cannabis, and (3) lack of knowledge surrounding medical cannabis (see Table 3.1). Additionally, participants explained that they were concerned about their lack of education regarding the therapeutic risks and benefits of prescribing medical cannabis. They specifically wanted information about the potential harms that medical cannabis had on neurocognitive development, interactions between medical cannabis and other medications, and the impact of medical cannabis on mental illness. Based on these results, Ng et al. (2021, p. E347) concluded that:

> Family physicians in our study were uncertain of the therapeutic potential of medical cannabis. The exception was the use of medical cannabis for chronic pain, particularly neuropathic pain, for which all participants thought the evidence supported effectiveness. Most physicians did not provide therapeutic cannabis to their patients and expressed uncertainty regarding its harms and appropriate use. Family physicians may benefit from guidance and education that address concerns they have surrounding medical cannabis.

Ng et al. (2022) published a study that outlined the attitudes and beliefs of pain physicians practising within the Greater Toronto and Hamilton area held about medical cannabis for managing chronic noncancer pain. Between February 2019 and December 2020, they interviewed 13 physicians. An analysis of the interview transcripts yielded three themes, which were: (1) evidence regarding medical cannabis, (2) medical cannabis as first-line therapy for chronic pain, and (3) barriers to accessing medical cannabis. They concluded that despite medical cannabis becoming

Table 3.1 Participant quotes supporting thematic analysis

Theme/ subtheme	Representative quote(s)
Reluctance to authorise medical cannabis	
Lack of evidence	I don't think most of the results of studies are that strong, they're not really well-designed studies for the most part … (MC001) … some studies show that it's really effective and some studies show that it's not very effective. I suspect we've reached the point where we're probably a little too liberal for the conditions we prescribe it for. (MC009)
Indications for therapeutic use	It's an okay adjunct, but it wouldn't be my first line for pain control at all. (MC002) … it's more of a second- or third-line treatment … certain patients will find it helpful. (MC004) There's very few things, if any, that I would go to medical cannabis as my first medication to treat. (MC008)
Discomfort with therapeutic use of cannabis	I'm not 100% comfortable prescribing it, I do feel it might be helpful for some conditions, but I'm just not sure of the entire process of how to go about prescribing it and monitoring its use. (MC001) I don't prescribe it at all, I usually refer it out to clinics who are specialized in that. (MC002) I would be happy if it went away, in terms of [the] physician's responsibility toward it. I do not want to be prescribing marijuana. (MC006)
Openness to emerging evidence	I think you have to keep an open mind, and you have to be attuned to what your patients are telling you … if you're not willing to listen to what patients are telling you about what they're using, and you don't present an unbiased front, then people aren't going to tell you what they're doing. (MC009) I think that we need to make sure we are providing our patients with access to evidence-based treatment and addressing any financial barriers and any stigma that may exist around particular treatments. I think we need to be careful of that when we are thinking about prescribing medical marijuana. (MC011)
Harms associated with the use of cannabis	
Effect on neurocognitive development	There is so much research saying that the brain is still changing and the reality is we don't know what happens to kids' brains when they take marijuana at the age of 15. And you know, I have so many patients who are young, who are like, "oh well now that is legalized for the age of 18, [and] I'm 14 and I'm so close, I'm sure it is fine." And I think the fact that legalization, especially at such a young age, gives the message to a lot of people that it's safe. (MC010)
Harms for older adults	Maybe sort of looking at long-term effects on older people. All the medications we prescribe, there are certain geriatric populations that take various medications so I just want to know if there's anything in particular or things to watch for. (MC002) What is the effect of adding a cannabis product into a geriatric population that tends to be already medically more complex and already on lots of other medications and have multiple comorbidities? So, what impact does that have potentially, on their quality of life, ability to continue to drive a car, ability to continue to take care of themselves, and maybe dependence issues. (MC009)

(continued)

Table 3.1 (continued)

Theme/ subtheme	Representative quote(s)
Exacerbation of mental illness	Our patients have mental health issues, ranging from depression to anxiety to schizophrenia, and you know, you worry about harms for people especially for people who have [mental] illnesses. (MC006) So some of the [symptoms] I've noticed so far have been an increase in anxiety, difficulty with sleep, even cases of potential psychosis. (MC007)
Concerns regarding cannabis clinics	Cannabis clinics are fairly easy to access for most of these [patients]. (MC004) I would, for the most part, send patients to marijuana [clinics]; there are a couple in Hamilton. Everyone wound up getting it. Most people that did had addiction issues and mental health issues. (MC006) I've had patients who've come in and were prescribed medical cannabis and I would be like "oh you are so young, did the people go through the risks with you?" and they were like "no not really" and so I think that concerns me because it seems like even depending on which cannabis clinic certain people are referred to, they are not necessarily being presented with both the pros and the cons. (MC010)
Lack of knowledge surrounding medical cannabis	
Inadequate training	I'd say my knowledge of [medical cannabis] is pretty average … average enough to know that I would refer someone else to [authorize] medical cannabis if I thought it would help. And also enough to say that it won't help with your kind of pain or your set of conditions. So, I would know enough about that, but in terms of dosing and things like that I am not as comfortable, but it's not something I sought to really train in. (MC002) I went to medical school 35 years ago, there was zero training about cannabis and anything I learned about cannabis has been through continuing education that consists of online courses and information, position statements and summaries, sessions at conferences… So, the training has been whatever I chose to participate in, there's nothing required of me. (MC005) We did have some lectures from physicians in residency, [and] we also read a few articles during that time as well. I definitely don't know all of the up-to-date research that's ongoing in marijuana, it's just the things that I'm coming across. (MC007)
Continuing education	I just don't know what the regulations are in terms of how that's monitored, so my [further] education would hopefully help me figure out where I can direct patients to, sort of more, reputable sources of marijuana once it's been prescribed. (MC002) Something that comes out from time to time, that would actually be very helpful to get updates about what's [new] with medical cannabis. (MC007)

(continued)

Table 3.1 (continued)

Theme/ subtheme	Representative quote(s)
Physician's role regarding cannabis	[Regarding medical cannabis], it is still not a prescription. A prescription includes the name of a substance, exactly what is in it, it includes a dosage, frequency, and duration. And it is dispensed by a pharmacist. None of those criteria are being fulfilled by cannabis. I am a little bit lost right now about what my form actually does for anyone. I think anyone and his dog can walk into a drug store and get whatever they want without approval from a physician. (MC004) Pretending that marijuana/cannabis is a prescription has been a joke … There is nothing about dosing or actual content; the traditional approach to making cannabis accessible really has just been to say this person has a medical condition and I believe this person may benefit from medical cannabis … Right now, it's very confusing why I have any role in making cannabis accessible to anyone. Whatever I write or say on a form does not decrease the cost of it. It does not make it funded, and it still does not provide any instructions that have to be followed … I would love to see [the] medical profession removed from the transaction completely and to make [cannabis] more like alcohol. (MC005)
Recreational v. medicinal cannabis	I'm not sure how [recreational] products are regulated and if they know how much THC or CBD is in it, so I am not sure if [using recreational cannabis for therapeutic purposes] would be a good idea. (MC003) I think it's still helpful … being prescribed medical cannabis because a lot of people are not sure what's the best time to take it for medical reasons. I still think there's a role for medical cannabis even if recreational cannabis is approved for use now. (MC004)

Note CBD cannabidiol, *THC* tetrahydrocannabinol
Source Ng et al. (2021, pp. E345–E346)

more commonly used in Canada, the physicians interviewed were unsure about the therapeutic benefits that medical cannabis gave people with chronic noncancer pain.

Rosenbaek et al. (2023) explored the amount of knowledge, attitudes, and experiences of prescribing medicinal cannabis among a sample of Danish general practitioners. From September 2018 to July 2019, they distributed an online survey to Danish physicians. Out of 112 general practitioners invited to participate, 427 (38.4%) completed the survey. Of those who completed the questionnaire, 37 (8.7%) had prescribed medicinal cannabis. Most had either a scant amount or no knowledge about medicinal cannabis (80.6%) and most had a negative view about prescribing medicinal cannabis (71.4%).

For the past seven years, medicinal cannabis have been available in Australia via prescription. Since it became possible to prescribe medicinal cannabis, there has been a significant rise in the number of prescriptions by general practitioners for this medication. Bawa et al. (2022) investigated Australian-based general practitioners' awareness, encounters, and opinions regarding medicinal cannabis. They also compared the results that they collected to those of their previous study that they conducted in 2017. Between November 2021 and February 2022, a total of 505 Australian-based general practitioners completed a 42-item online questionnaire, that they modified from their 2017 study. From this survey, they allocated the collected data into the following five categories:

1. medicinal cannabis prescribing experiences,
2. indications for medicinal cannabis usage,
3. attitudes of general practitioners towards prescribing medicinal cannabis,
4. perceived knowledge of general practitioners about medicinal cannabis, and
5. concerns that general practitioners had about medicinal cannabis.

Each of these five categories are elaborated below.

Medicinal cannabis prescribing experiences

In the previous three months before completing their online survey, most participants ($n = 431$ out of 505, 85.3%) reported that they had encountered at least one inquiry from a patient about prescribing medicinal cannabis. Additionally, among those that had received patient inquiries about prescribing medicinal cannabis, most participants ($n = 280$ out of 505, 55.4%) received between one to four inquiries. Despite most participants reported receiving such inquiries, just more than half ($n = 264$ out of 505, 52.3%) reported that they felt comfortable discussing with their patients the risks and benefits associated with them using medicinal cannabis (Bawa et al., 2022).

Slightly more than one-fifth of all general practitioners who completed Bawa et al.'s online survey ($n = 110$ out of 505, 21.8%) had prescribed medicinal cannabis during their medical careers. These respondents were termed *'prescribers'*. During the three months prior to completing Bawa et al.'s online survey, more than half of all prescribers ($n = 67$ out of 110, 60%) had issued between one to nine medicinal cannabis prescriptions for their patients. Most of these prescriptions were new instead of being repeat prescriptions ($n = 67$ out of 110, 60.9%). Additionally, the SAS-B pathway was predominantly used ($n = 92$ out of 110, 83.6%). Finally, most prescribers held the belief that cannabis should *'only'* be legally accessible for medicinal purposes instead for both medicinal and recreational purposes ($n = 72$ out of 110, 65.5%) (Bawa et al., 2022).

The prescribers reported that they had prescribed a diverse variety of distinct medicinal cannabis products, ranging from only one product ($n = 36$ out of 110, 32.7%) to more than five products ($n = 17$ out of 110, 15.4%). Most prescribers indicated that they preferred prescribing medicinal cannabis products that were predominantly composed of CBD ($n = 79$ out of 110, 71.8%). Conversely, a minority of prescribers wrote prescriptions for products that predominantly contained THC ($n = 30$ out of 110, 27.3%). Additionally, a significant number of prescribers had wrote for their patient's prescription for medicinal cannabis products that contained a combination of THC and CBD ($n = 78$ out of 110, 70.9%). Finally, most prescribers cited oil formulations ($n = 104$ out of 110, 94.5%), followed by flower (also known as *'flos'* or *'plant material'*) ($n = 29$ out of 110, 26.4%) and capsules ($n = 12$ out of 110, 10.9%) in response to being asked about the *'forms'* of medicinal cannabis that they had prescribed to their patients (Bawa et al., 2022).

Indications for medicinal cannabis usage

Those who were prescribers, who constituted 21.8% (n = 110 out of 505) of the entire sample, predominantly prescribed medicinal cannabis for patients with chronic noncancer pain (n = 102 out of 110, 92.7%), followed by anxiety (n = 72 out of 110, 65.5%) and neuropathic pain (n = 68 out of 110, 61.8%). However, considering prescribers and non-prescribers combined (n = 505), medicinal cannabis for patients in end-of-life/palliative care (n = 468 out of 505, 92.7%) was predominantly endorsed. In contrast only a few respondents endorsed medicinal cannabis for treating depression (n = 188 out of 505, 37.2%) (see Fig. 3.1) (Bawa et al., 2022).

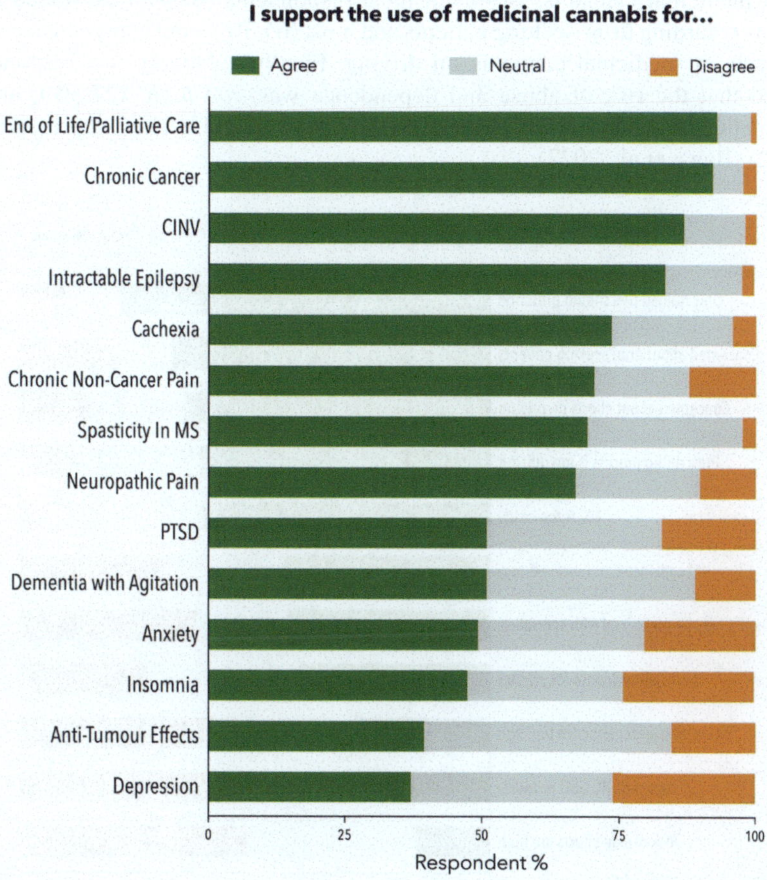

Fig. 3.1 Extent to which general practitioners support use of medicinal cannabis to treat certain conditions (n = 505). *CINV* chemotherapy-induced nausea and vomiting; *MS* multiple sclerosis; *PTSD* post-traumatic stress disorder. *Source* Bawa et al. (2022, p. 4)

Attitudes of general practitioners towards prescribing medicinal cannabis

Most respondents who completed Bawa et al.'s study expressed that they had challenges in navigating the prescribing process, with 62% of them reporting difficulties. Additionally, 61.4% expressed the view that medicinal cannabis products were too costly. A substantial proportion (79%) believed that general practitioners should undergo specific training so that they could help prescribe medicinal cannabis. However, a few respondents (42.8%) supported the notion that general practitioners should only prescribe medicinal cannabis with specialist support. There was limited support for making CBD products available over the counter in pharmacies (23.8%). Additionally, few respondents (43.8%) held doubts about the effectiveness of medicinal cannabis. However, most respondents (67.9%) expressed some concerns regarding drug-seeking patients and most (65.3%) were apprehensive about the effects of medicinal cannabis on driving. Finally, relatively few respondents believed that the risk of abuse and dependence was *'too high'* (27.3%), and an even smaller percentage (15.6%) believed the risk of side effects was excessive (see Fig. 3.2) (Bawa et al., 2022).

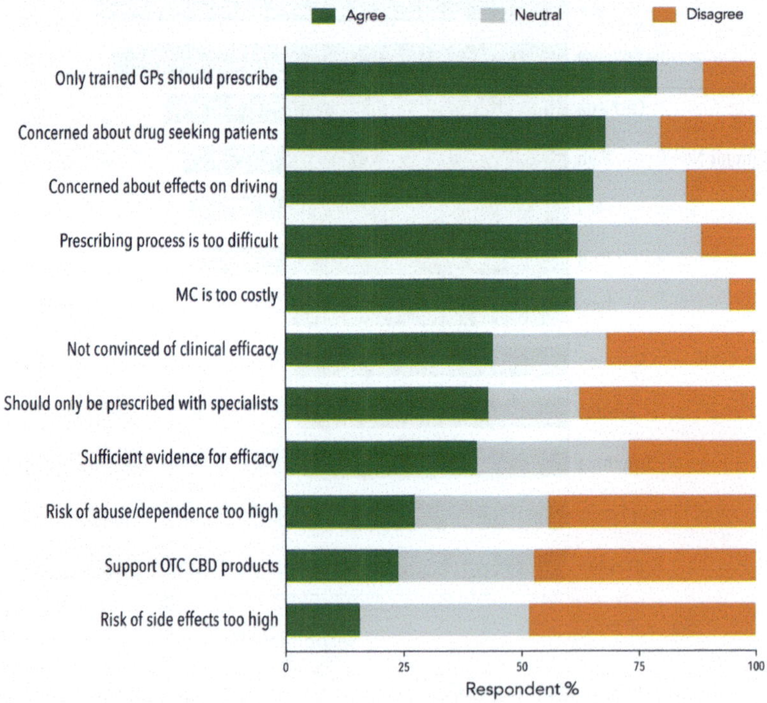

Fig. 3.2 Attitudes towards, and perceptions of, medicinal cannabis prescribing and use ($n = 505$). *GP* general practitioner; *MC* medicinal cannabis; *CBD* cannabidiol; *OTC* over the counter. *Source* Bawa et al. (2022, p. 5)

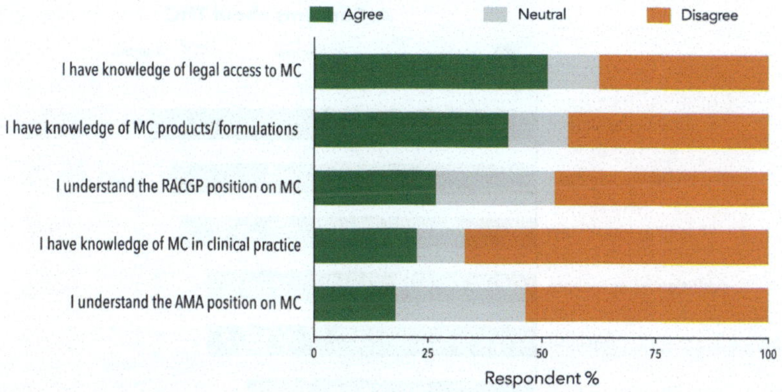

Fig. 3.3 Perceived knowledge of medicinal cannabis as expressed by general practitioners (n = 505). *AMA* Australian Medical Association; *RACGP* Royal Australian college of general practitioners; *MC* medicinal cannabis. *Source* Bawa et al. (2022, p. 6)

Perceived knowledge of general practitioners about medicinal cannabis

A small percentage of respondents (22.6%) believed that they possessed an adequate level of knowledge about the use of medicinal cannabis in clinical environments. Just more than half of respondents were knowledgeable about how to assist patients in accessing medicinal cannabis (51.1%) and less than half were aware of the available products and their formulations (42.6%). As expected, compared to non-prescribers, those who prescribed medicinal cannabis expressed a greater perceived level of knowledge about medicinal cannabis. Finally, awareness of the stated positions of the Australian Medical Association (AMA) and the Royal Australian College of General Practitioners (RACGP) on medicinal cannabis was limited among participants, with only 18% being aware of the AMA's stance and 26.7% were aware of the RACGP's position (see Fig. 3.3) (Bawa et al., 2022).

Concerns that general practitioners had about medicinal cannabis

Regarding products containing THC, participants expressed concerns about various consequences of medicinal cannabis usage, including driving impairment (75.2%), impact on the developing brain (71.1%), cognitive impairment (69.1%), addiction and dependence (64.4%), and psychosis (64%). However, the participants' stance on the concern of weight gain was mostly neutral, with 56.8% expressing neutrality, 28.1% expressing agreement, and 15% expressing disagreement (see Fig. 3.4, Panel A) (Bawa et al., 2022).

Regarding CBD products, participants expressed concerns about the potential effects of medicinal cannabis usage on the developing brain (55.4%) and possible interactions with other medications (51.9%). Additionally, despite the limited evidence supporting such apprehensions, medicinal cannabis usage causing driving impairments (50.7%) and worries about developing an addiction or dependence on

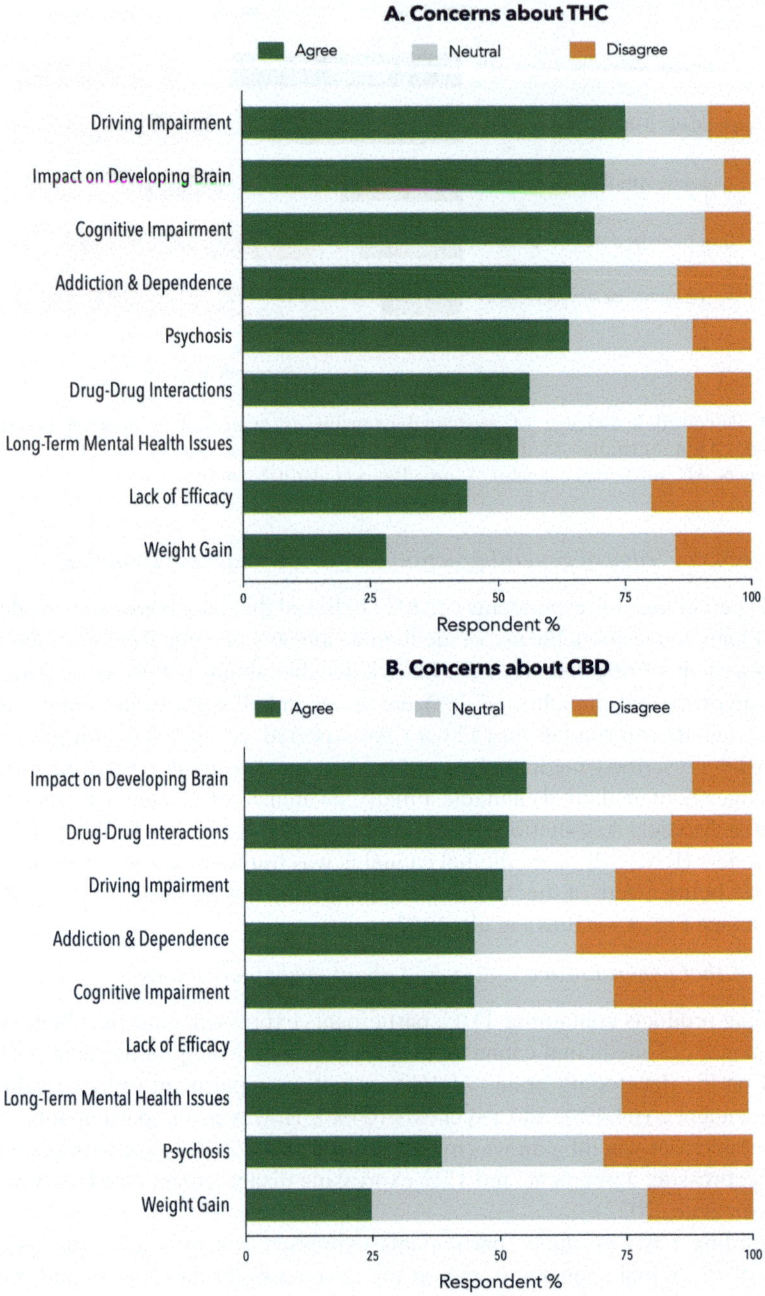

Fig. 3.4 Concerns around safety and efficacy of THC and CBD products ($n = 505$). *Notes* Panel A concerns around the safety and efficacy of THC products ($n = 505$). Panel B concerns around the safety and efficacy of CBD products ($n = 505$). Numbers show percentage of general practitioners ($n = 505$) endorsing agreement, disagreement, and neutrality around specific concerns. *Source* Bawa et al. (2022, p. 7)

medicinal cannabis (45.1%) were also cited as significant concerns (see Fig. 3.4, Panel B) (Bawa et al., 2022).

Participants were questioned about if medicinal cannabis was perceived to be more hazardous than commonly prescribed medications. In general, most participants disagreed that medicinal cannabis was more hazardous than opioids (64.4%), benzodiazepines (63.8%), and chemotherapy drugs (57%). Additionally, although a notable proportion expressed neutrality regarding these latter companions, a minority of participants tended to disagree that medicinal cannabis was more hazardous than antipsychotics (47.1%), antidepressants (40.4%), and statins (34.9%) (see Fig. 3.5) (Bawa et al., 2022).

Based on their results, Bawa et al. explained that since 2017 there has been an increased acceptance among general practitioners of medicinal cannabis as a treatment option. Nevertheless, there is a distinct requirement for enhanced training and education of general practitioners regarding cannabis-based medicines to foster a greater number of proficient prescribers within the medical community. In conclusion, Bawa et al. (2022, p. 9) concluded that:

> There is accelerating demand for MC [medicinal cannabis] products in Australia, in line with global trends. GPs [General Practitioners] are well positioned to assist in the safe and efficacious use of cannabis-based medicines in the community. Training around MC is required to address the long-standing concerns of GPs around knowledge and confidence in this area. Findings from this study can be used to develop educational initiatives and promote best practice. Australia has the potential to act as exemplar for other countries in guiding

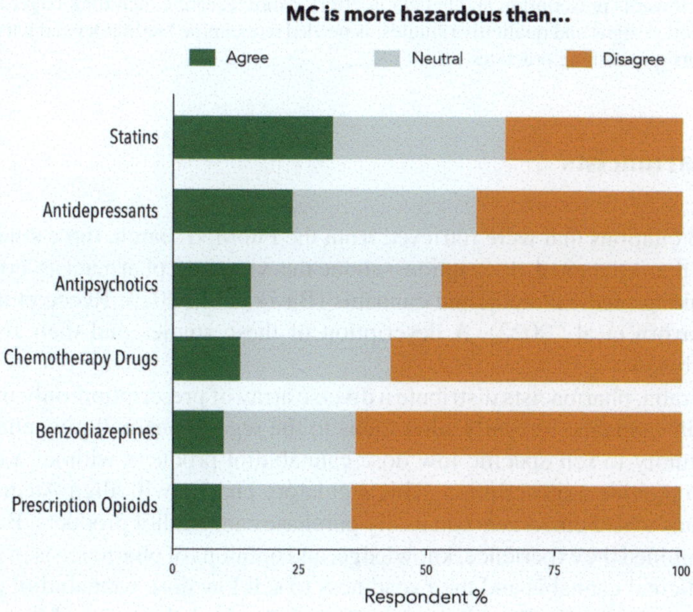

Fig. 3.5 General Practitioners tended to disagree that medicinal cannabis products were 'more hazardous' than commonly prescribed medications ($n = 505$). *Source* Bawa et al. (2022, p. 8)

> high quality MC prescribing and product utilisation in a government-regulated model. Many countries, such as the United Kingdom, face similar access challenges as those of Australia but are yet to utilise GPs as independent MC prescribers, limiting MC prescribing approvals to specialists only.

Despite their authority to prescribe medical cannabis, general practitioners believe that they do not have enough evidence based knowledge or confidence to prescribe medical cannabis products to their patients. Rønne et al. (2021) published a literature review about the experiences, attitudes, and beliefs of hospital physicians and general practitioners about medical cannabis. They examined 21 studies that were sourced from PubMed, Scopus, EMBASE, and the Cochrane Library (see Appendix E). They discovered that medical staff from a diverse variety of specialities encountered patient demands for medical cannabis. Those general practitioners and hospital physicians who prescribed medical cannabis were more convinced of its benefits and were less worried about its adverse effects. Finally, most studies showed that physicians had a limited amount of knowledge about the beneficial and adverse effects of medical cannabis and how to advise patients about these benefits and shortcomings. They concluded that:

> hospital physicians and GPs in various specialties experience inquiries about medical cannabis from their patients, and to some extent show openness to provide it, although there was a wide gap between studies in terms of willingness to provide. Most hospital physicians' and GPs' experience a lack of knowledge of beneficial effects, adverse effects and of how to advise patients. Hence, hospital physicians' and GPs' experiences with prescribing medical cannabis, and their knowledge as well as their specialty, may be associated with their attitudes towards prescription and beliefs in effect. More research, including larger studies with cohort designs and qualitative studies, is needed to examine facilitators and barriers to physicians' prescribing practices.

3.2 Pharmacists

Of the 683 citations that were retrieved from the PubMed search, three studies were identified that contained descriptions about the views of pharmacists concerning patients taking medical/medicinal cannabis (Bawa et al., 2023; Reece et al., 2021; Sabmeethavorn et al., 2022). A description of these studies and their results are presented below.

In Australia, pharmacists distribute a diverse array of prescription-only medicines that contain cannabis. Recently, alterations to the regulations will give pharmacists the opportunity to sell specific low dose cannabidiol products without a customer needing to provide a prescription. This regulatory change will align Australia with other nations where customers can easily purchase cannabidiol products. Bawa et al. (2023) examined the experience, knowledge, and opinions of pharmacists in Australia about medicinal cannabis and their readiness to sell low dose cannabidiol products. Based on prior surveys of health professionals, Bawa et al. designed a 51-item online questionnaire to achieve their study's objectives. From May to December 2021, pharmacists in Australia were invited to complete the 51-item online questionnaire.

They were recruited primarily from professional pharmacy organisations. Surveys were deemed as valid if the respondent completed the section about the demographic characteristics and at least one additional section. Out of the 272 survey attempts, 217 respondents were judged to be valid for inclusion in the final dataset. The data collected was catalogued into the following topics:

- Pharmacists' experience with the supply of medicinal cannabis products,
- Pharmacists' attitudes towards the supply of medicinal cannabis products,
- Knowledge about medicinal cannabis products, and
- Pharmacists' professional education needs (Bawa et al., 2023).

The results about these topics are now presented.

Pharmacists' experiences with the supply of medicinal cannabis products

During their careers, most respondents who completed the online survey (n = 130 out of 217, 60%) had sold at least one cannabis product that required a prescription. Two months before completing this survey, 39.2% (n = 85 out of 217) had dispensed medicinal cannabis, and among this subset of the sample, a substantial minority (n = 66 out of 217, 77.6%) had dispensed from one to nine prescriptions for medicinal cannabis. A minority of respondents (n = 10 out of 217, 4.6%) had dispensed 20 or more medicinal cannabis prescriptions in the two months before completing the survey. Most respondents (n = 123 out of 217, 56.7%) recalled that they had encountered an increase in the number of inquiries about medicinal cannabis over the previous three months. Furthermore, most respondents (n = 127 out of 217, 58.5%) had received at least one inquiry about medicinal cannabis in the last two weeks (Bawa et al., 2023).

Irrespective of their previous involvement in supplying medicinal cannabis, slightly more than half of the respondents (n = 117 out of 217, 53.9%) felt *'comfortable supplying medicinal cannabis products and wised to do so in future'*. The remaining respondents (n = 100 out of 217, 46.1%) indicated feeling:

- neither comfortable nor uncomfortable (n = 43 out of 217, 19.8%),
- not comfortable supplying medicinal cannabis products now but interested in doing so in future (n = 44 out of 217, 20.3%), or
- not comfortable supplying medicinal cannabis products and not wishing to do so in future (n = 13 out of 217, 6%) (Bawa et al., 2023).

Respondents who had dispensed medicinal cannabis products (n = 130 out of 217, 60%) were provided with a list of common medical conditions and were asked to identify the top three for which they believed medicinal cannabis was most prescribed based on their professional experience. The primary condition identified was noncancer pain (n = 120 out of 217, 55.3%), followed by anxiety (n = 63 out of 217, 29%), neuropathic pain (n = 57 out of 217, 26.3%), chronic cancer pain (n = 46 out of 217, 21.2%), insomnia (n = 33 out of 217, 15.2%), childhood epilepsy (n = 30 out of 217, 13.8%), spasticity (n = 20 out of 217, 9.2%), 'other' (6.9%), depression (n 14 out of 217, 6.5%), and 'unsure' (n = 1 out of 217, 0.5%) (Bawa et al., 2023).

Pharmacists' attitudes towards the supply of medicinal cannabis products

Out of the 217 respondents who completed the survey, 201 respondents provided their attitude towards selling medicinal cannabis and *Pharmacist Only* CBD products. Most respondents ($n = 136$ out of 201, 67.7%) expressed *'agreement'* that community pharmacies selling medicinal cannabis represents a *'positive'* development for the pharmacy profession. This sentiment persisted even though most respondents ($n = 140$ out of 201, 69.6%) acknowledged an existing stigma associated with the usage of medicinal cannabis products. Most respondents ($n = 118$ out of 201, 58.7%) were in favour of providing Pharmacist Only CBD products for eligible patients. However, a minority of respondents (39.3%) believed that they felt that they could confidently answer customers' enquiries about medicinal cannabis products. Few respondents ($n = 57$ out of 201, 28.4%) understood recent scheduling changes that impacted Pharmacy Only CBD products. Few respondents ($n = 65$ out of 201, 32.4%) were aware of the current variety of medicinal cannabis products or their formulations. Among respondents were different opinions about the willingness of general practitioners to prescribe medicinal cannabis products to their patients and whether they should determine the suitability of Pharmacist Only CBD products for patients (see Fig. 3.6) (Bawa et al., 2023).

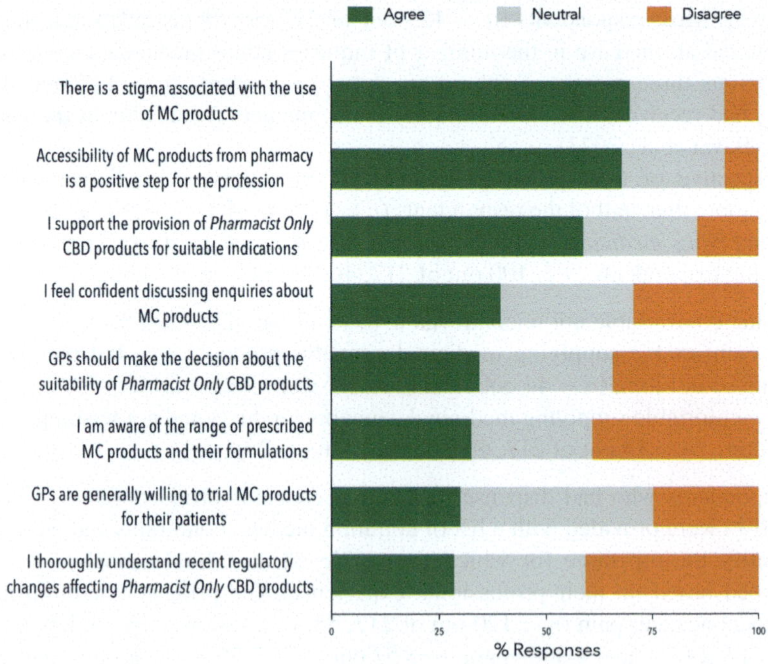

Fig. 3.6 Pharmacists' responses to statements on various aspects of supply of medicinal cannabis and 'Pharmacist Only' CBD products, $n = 201$, valid percentage. *MC* medicinal cannabis. *Source* Bawa et al. (2023, p. 379)

All respondents ($n = 217$) were given a list of potential obstacles and were asked to select all options that they believed would have an impact on the availability of Pharmacist Only CBD products. The three barriers that were most cited were:

- insufficient training and resources for pharmacists and staff ($n = 133$ out of 217, 61.3%),
- concerns related to patient safety, such as the potential for misuse, abuse, or diversion ($n = 115$ out of 217, 53%), and
- a demand for Pharmacist Only CBD products without the product being available ($n = 114$ out of 217, 52.5%) (see Fig. 3.7) (Bawa et al., 2023).

Respondents were provided with a list of plausible advantages of using Pharmacist Only CBD products. Respondents were allowed to select as many options as they wanted. The three most selected options were:

- enhanced access to medicinal cannabis products for patients ($n = 122$ out of 217, 56.2%),
- continuity of care ($n = 103$ out of 217, 47.5%), and
- a decreased burden on the healthcare system ($n = 98$ out of 217, 45.2%) (see Fig. 3.8) (Bawa et al., 2023).

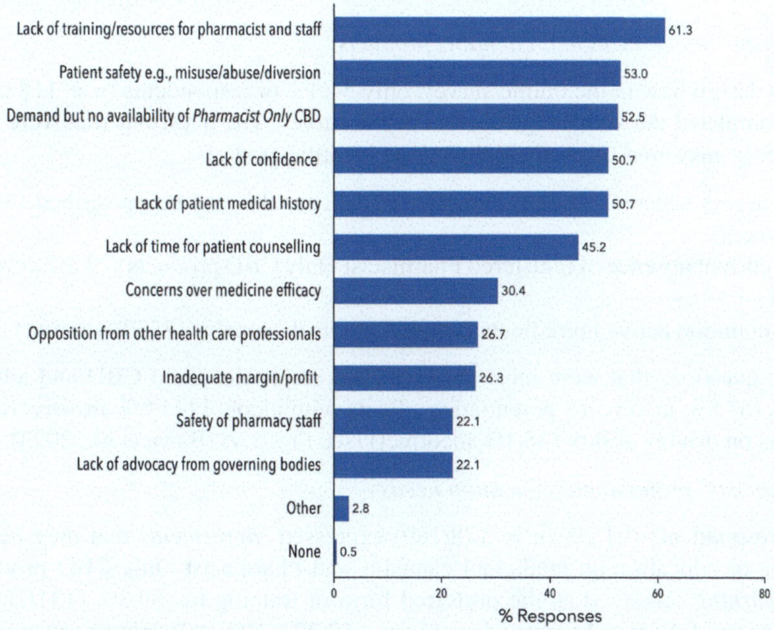

Fig. 3.7 Pharmacists' perceived barriers around implementation of 'Pharmacist Only' CBD products. *Notes* Pharmacists ($n = 217$) were instructed to select all applicable options. Each bar represents % of total respondents ($n = 217$) who selected this option. *MC* medicinal cannabis. *Source* Bawa et al. (2023, p. 380)

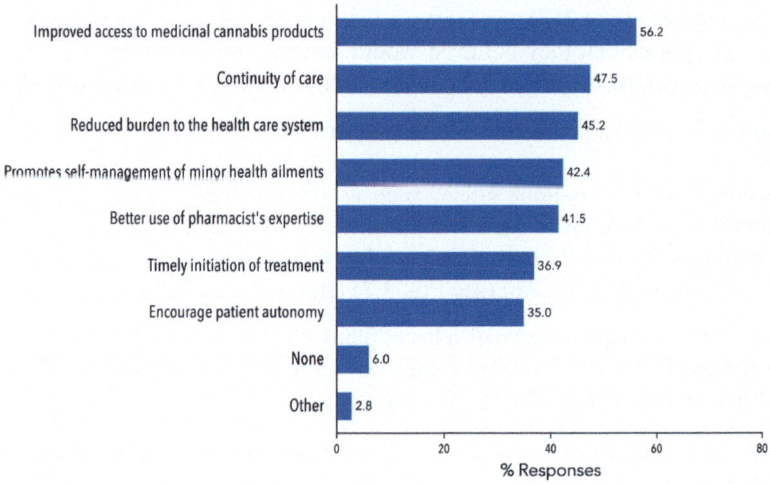

Fig. 3.8 Pharmacists' perceived benefits around implementation of pharmacist only CBD products. *Notes* Pharmacists ($n = 217$) were instructed to select all applicable options. Each bar represents % of total respondents ($n = 217$) who selected this option. *MC* medicinal cannabis. *Source* Bawa et al. (2023, p. 381)

Knowledge about medicinal cannabis products

Due to design flaw in the online survey, only 54.4% of respondents ($n = 118$ out of 217) completed the knowledge section of the survey. The questions that were most frequently answered correctly included the identification of:

- the access schemes through which medical cannabis can be prescribed (81.9% correct),
- the current absence of registered Pharmacist Only CBD products (78.8% correct), and
- the common active ingredients found in medical cannabis (73.7% correct).

The questions that were most answered incorrectly involved CBD and adverse effects (67.8% incorrect), potentiating effects with alcohol (41.5% incorrect), and impacts on driving ability (38.1% incorrect) (see Fig. 3.9) (Bawa et al., 2023).

Pharmacists' professional education needs

Most respondents (94.2%, $n = 178/189$) expressed *'agreement'* that they needed training or education on medicinal cannabis and Pharmacist Only CBD products. *'Self-learning'* emerged as the preferred form of training for 69.3% (131/189) of participants, followed by virtual webinars (57.7%, 109/189), pharmacy journals (47.0%, 89/189), and in-person workshops (33.3%, 63/189). However, slightly more than half of the respondents (54.5%, 103/189) *'disagreed'* that they received adequate support and information on medicinal cannabis and Pharmacist Only CBD products from their professional pharmacy organisations (Bawa et al., 2023).

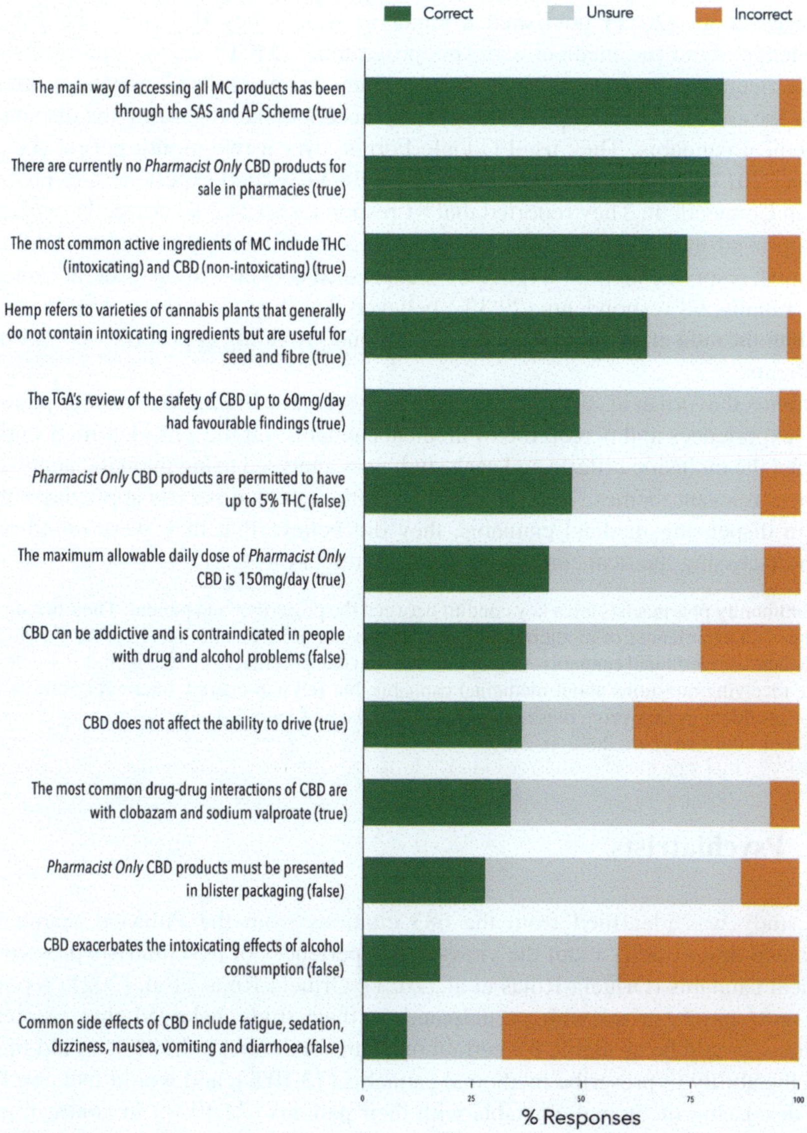

Fig. 3.9 Knowledge of pharmacists around cannabis-based medicines. *Notes* Figure shows percentage for each question that were answered correctly, incorrectly or as 'unsure' by pharmacists, $n = 118$, valid percentage. Correct answers provided after each question. *MC* medicinal cannabis; *SAS* special access scheme; *AP Scheme* authorised prescriber scheme; *THC* tetrahydrocannabinol; *CBD* cannabidiol; *TGA* therapeutic goods administration. *Source* Bawa et al. (2023, p. 382)

Reece et al. (2021) published a study in which they described the gaps in knowledge about the medical cannabis programme (MCP) among pharmacists in Connecticut, the impact of MCP on pharmacy practices in Connecticut, and to assess the concerns among pharmacists in Connecticut had regarding the dispensing of medical cannabis. They used Google Forms, over a two-month period (i.e., 15 October 2017–15 December 2017), to collect the views and experiences of pharmacists in Connecticut. They reported that 81 respondents (24.2%) correctly explained the approved maximum monthly dosage of 2.5 oz of medical cannabis. Additionally, most respondents ($n = 243$, 72.5%) expressed concerns about federal cannabis laws. Finally, 98 respondents (29.3%) believed that they were competent in understanding the side effects of medical cannabis and providing appropriate counselling to patients.

Sabmeethavorn et al.'s (2022) published a systematic literature review of pharmacists' experiences and perception of medical cannabis. Of the 278 identified studies, five met the inclusion criteria and each study was analysed using thematic analysis to discover relevant themes. They reported that although pharmacists appreciated their role in dispensing medical cannabis, they did believe that they were uninformed when discussing medical cannabis to their customers.

> Community pharmacists are a key conduit between the prescriber and patient. Their perceptions and experiences of medicinal cannabis dispensing are crucial in meeting the growing demand for medicinal cannabis. This review showed that pharmacists in the included articles are receiving questions about medicinal cannabis, but felt unprepared, uncomfortable, and not confident in answering these questions, with a lack of knowledge as the primary driver. (Sabmeethavorn et al., 2022, p. 212)

3.3 Psychiatrists

One study was identified from the 683 citations from the PubMed search that contained descriptions about the views and experiences of psychiatrists prescribing medical cannabis (Orjuela-Rojas et al., 2021). Orjuela-Rojas et al. (2021) reported that most psychiatrists who participated in their study believed that medicinal cannabis should be available for certain medical conditions (82.10%), would like to have the ability to prescribe medicinal cannabis (73.10%), and would feel comfortable discussing medicinal cannabis with their patients (72.40%). In contrast, most psychiatrists did not know how to legally access medicinal cannabis medications for their patients (66.20%) and most did not know the current status of the legislation regarding medicinal cannabis (46.90%).

3.4 Patients

Unlike the previous chapter, that described the therapeutic benefits that medial cannabis gave patients, this section describes the non-therapeutic benefits and challenges patients experienced while using medical cannabis. Examples of non-therapeutic benefits include administrative barriers, negative social judgements, prohibitive costs, legal concerns, and a lack of information or medical support. In contrast, examples of non-therapeutic benefits include medical cannabis being chapter than other medications and medical professionals being knowledgeable about medical cannabis.

An examination of the 683 studies retrieved from the PubMed search revealed three that contained descriptions about the non-therapeutic experiences of patients using medical cannabis (Erridge et al., 2023; Garcia-Romeu et al., 2022; Gliksberg et al., 2023). A description of these studies and their results are outlined below.

Erridge et al. (2023) examined the research priorities of patients taking medical cannabis in the United Kingdom. From December 2021 to February 2022, patients taking medical cannabis for health conditions were invited to disclose their views and experiences of medical cannabis in focus groups. The researchers conducted an inductive thematic analysis of the participants' responses to derive their insights. Additionally, participants also completed a ranking exercise whereby they assigned ten tokens (with each token representing a £1 million pounds of public funding) to competing research priorities. In total, 30 patients taking medical cannabis were divided into one of three focus groups. A collection of research priorities were identified, which were adverse events, comparing cannabis-based medicinal products, health conditions, pharmacology of cannabis, healthcare professionals' attitudes, agriculture and manufacturing, and learning about the cannabis plant (see Table 3.2). Collectively, participants wanted most funding to be allocated to studying the cannabis plant (5.7%) and participants prioritised funding research about medical cannabis treating chronic pain (4%).

Garcia-Romeu et al. (2022) explored the self-perceptions of the benefits and challenges that patients taking medical cannabis experience. They distributed an anonymous online survey in which the participants recorded their demographics, health information, and open-ended responses about their perceptions, motivations, and experience of taking medical cannabis. All qualitative responses were thematically analysed. Participants often used medicinal cannabis to treat neurological disorders (38%) or pain (25%). Believing that traditional medical treatments were ineffective and/or had intolerable side effects (51%), positive media and scientific portrayals that medicinal cannabis is safe and effective (29%) or being regarded as a *'natural'* treatment compared to pharmaceuticals (21%) were the primary motivators for using medicinal cannabis. Most respondents (77%) reported that medicinal cannabis had positive effects, such as improvements in physical functioning (51%), mental health (29%), and quality of life (14%). In contrast, the setbacks of medicinal cannabis disclosed by the recipients included unwanted side effects (16%), lack of medical

Table 3.2 Allocation of counters according to research priorities by focus group participants

Priorities	Total (*n*)	Proportion of funding (%)
Research about		
The cannabis plant	17	5.7
The endocannabinoid system	16	5.3
Specific cannabinoids	6	2.0
Specific terpenes	5	1.7
Specific flavonoids	3	1.0
Whole plant extract/flower	2	0.7
Over the counter CBD oils/edibles	5	1.7
Targeted research on strains	1	0.3
Growing techniques and production	2	0.7
Research about medical cannabis and specific conditions		
Chronic pain	12	4.0
Fibromyalgia	4	1.3
Anxiety	10	3.3
Epilepsy	1	0.3
Post-traumatic stress disorder	10	3.3
Menopause	3	1.0
Sleep disorders and insomnia	2	0.7
Hypertension	1	0.3
Addiction disorders	1	0.3
Autistic spectrum disorder	4	1.3
Schizophrenia	3	1.0
Myalgic encephalomyelitis	2	0.7
Attention-deficit hyperactivity disorder	4	1.3
Migraine	1	0.3
Cancer	1	0.3
Research that uses the following methods		
Randomised controlled trials	16	5.3
Real-world evidence	15	5.0
Research that aims to		
Understand how chemicals from the cannabis plant work in the body	8	2.7
Discover other chemicals from the cannabis plant	1	0.3
Understand the effect of medical cannabis on specific symptoms	26	8.7
Understand the effect of medical cannabis on quality of life	20	6.7
Understand the cost-effectiveness of medical cannabis as a treatment option	13	4.3

(continued)

Table 3.2 (continued)

Priorities	Total (*n*)	Proportion of funding (%)
Understand the adverse effects of medical cannabis	4	1.3
Interactions with different medications	1	0.3
How to use the medication/dose control	1	0.3
Delivery methods	1	0.3
Research that aims to		
Understand the barriers to accessing medical cannabis	16	5.3
Understand the knowledge of medical cannabis among healthcare professionals	20	6.7
Understand the stigma in society of medical cannabis patients	20	6.7
The effects of medical cannabis on driving and on ability to perform certain jobs	20	6.7
Understand the knowledge of medical cannabis among the criminal justice system	2	0.7
The understanding of medical cannabis by the press	1	0.3

Notes CBD cannabidiol. Each counter was assigned an equivalent monetary value of £1 million GBP. Each participant held a total of ten counters. Each participant assigned all their counters during this task. Participants could not divide their counters into smaller proportions but could allocate more than one counter to each priority
Source Erridge et al. (2023, p. 6)

support and information about medicinal cannabis (16%), prohibitive costs (12%), and legal concerns (10%) (see Table 3.3).

Gliksberg et al. (2023) examined eight studies about patients' experiences of medicinal cannabis. The studies were retrieved from either PubMed, PsycINFO, and EMBASE. They identified six main themes from the examined literature, which were: (1) medicinal cannabis approval, (2) administrative barriers, (3) social perceptions, (4) misuse and widespread effect of medicinal cannabis, (5) adverse effects of medicinal cannabis, and (6) dependence or addiction to medicinal cannabis. They concluded that:

> Results from this review indicate that actions should be taken to allow more accessible process of MC approval and acquisition by reducing administrative barriers to standardised treatment. In addition, health professionals should be aware of the stigma concerning MC use and its effect on patients' experience and behaviours and work towards decreasing its effect. Finally, physicians, nurses and mental health professionals should maintain close attention to patients' risk for developing of abuse and addiction, and decrease the risk for deviations or negative consequences of MC treatment. (Gliksberg et al., 2023, p. 5615)

Table 3.3 Major themes and subthemes identified from participants' open-ended responses and observed prevalence among study sample ($N = 808$)

Major themes/subthemes	*n*, %
Cannabis products	399, 49%
Factors driving use	538, 67%
Medical conditions	432, 53%
Traditional treatments ineffective/intolerable	415, 51%
Positive scientific or media portrayals	234, 29%
Prefer natural products	170, 21%
Recommended by trusted parties	136, 17%
Last resort	127, 16%
Curiosity or other factors	127, 16%
Good effects	624, 77%
Physical symptom improvements	446, 55%
Mental health improvements	232, 29%
QOL improvements	116, 14%
Reduced medications or healthcare utilisation	93, 12%
Too early or unsure	127, 16%
Issues or problems	330, 41%
Side effects	130, 16%
Lack of information or support	127, 16%
High cost	97; 12%
Too early or unsure	96, 12%
Legal concerns	81, 10%
Difficult to access	54, 7%
Not fully effective	46, 6%
Social stigma	31, 4%
Other concerns	29, 4%

Notes QOL quality of life
Source Garcia-Romeu et al. (2022, p. 4)

3.5 Conclusion

This chapter presented the literature about the views, experiences, and beliefs that healthcare professionals held about prescribing medical/medicinal cannabis and patients taking this medication. It was discovered that most healthcare professionals within several studies lacked training about recommending or prescribing medical/medicinal cannabis and did not know how to help patients legally access medical/medicinal cannabis. From a patient perspective, within several studies patients who were prescribed medical/medicinal cannabis described administrative and legal barriers that prevented them from accessing this medication.

References

Adler, L., Zacay, G., Schonmann, Y., Azuri, J., Yehoshua, I., Vinker, S., Shani, M., Heymann, A. D., & Hoffman, R. (2022). Primary care physicians' attitudes and knowledge regarding medical cannabis and willingness to prescribe it: The Israeli experience. *Family Practice, 39*(1), 59–64. https://doi.org/10.1093/fampra/cmab108

Alharbi, F. F., Alqahtani, T. M., Alzamil, A. M., Alharbi, N. H., & Masud, N. (2023). Knowledge, perception, and beliefs of Saudi physicians at King Abdulaziz Medical City, Riyadh related to medical cannabis: Literature review and a cross-sectional survey. *Journal of Family Medicine and Primary Care, 12*(3), 536–544. https://doi.org/10.4103/jfmpc.jfmpc_1856_22

Bawa, Z., McCartney, D., Manocha, R., & McGregor, I. S. (2022). Knowledge, experiences, and attitudes of Australian general practitioners towards medicinal cannabis: A 2021–2022 survey. *BMC Primary Care, 23*(1), 330. https://doi.org/10.1186/s12875-022-01946-x

Bawa, Z., Saini, B., McCartney, D., Bedoya-Pérez, M., McLachlan, A. J., & McGregor, I. S. (2023). A cross-sectional survey exploring the knowledge, experiences and attitudes of Australian pharmacists toward medicinal cannabis. *International Journal of Clinical Pharmacy, 45*(2), 375–386. https://doi.org/10.1007/s11096-022-01519-z

Bui, K., Worster, B., Ryan, J., Pant, S., & Kelly, E. L. (2023). Physicians' perspectives on their training for and role within Pennsylvania's medical cannabis program. *Journal of the American Board of Family Medicine, 36*(4), 670–681. https://doi.org/10.3122/jabfm.2022.220304R1

Cheng, K. Y. C., Harnett, J. E., Davis, S. R., Eassey, D., Law, S., & Smith, L. (2022). Healthcare professionals' perspectives on the use of medicinal cannabis to manage chronic pain: A systematic search and narrative review. *Pain Practice: The Official Journal of World Institute of Pain, 22*(8), 718–732. https://doi.org/10.1111/papr.13161

Dassieu, L., Paul-Savoie, E., Develay, É., Villela Guilhon, A. C., Guénette, L., Perreault, K., Beaudry, H., Dupuis, L., Audet, C., & Lacasse, A. (2023). Experiences and perceptions of medical cannabis among people living with chronic pain and community pharmacists: A qualitative study in Canada. *Canadian Journal of Pain, 7*(1), 2258537. https://doi.org/10.1080/24740527.2023.2258537

Erridge, S., Olsson, F., & Sodergren, M. H. (2023). Patient priorities for research: A focus group study of UK medical cannabis patients. *Complementary Therapies in Clinical Practice, 50*, 101693. https://doi.org/10.1016/j.ctcp.2022.101693

Garcia-Romeu, A., Elmore, J., Mayhugh, R. E., Schlienz, N. J., Martin, E. L., Strickland, J. C., Bonn-Miller, M., Jackson, H., & Vandrey, R. (2022). Online survey of medicinal cannabis users: Qualitative analysis of patient-level data. *Frontiers in Pharmacology, 13*, 965535. https://doi.org/10.3389/fphar.2022.965535

Gliksberg, O., Kushnir, T., Sznitman, S. R., Lev-Ran, S., Brill, S., Amit, B. H., & Feingold, D. (2023). Negative experiences of patients using medicinal cannabis: A systematic review of qualitative studies. *Journal of Clinical Nursing, 32*(17–18), 5607–5618. https://doi.org/10.1111/jocn.16653

Gunning, M., Rotenberg, A. D., Kelly, L. E., Crooks, B., Oberoi, S., Rapoport, A. L., Rassekh, S. R., & Illes, J. (2022). Clinician views on and ethics priorities for authorizing medical cannabis in the care of children and youth in Canada: A qualitative study. *CMAJ Open, 10*(1), E196–E202. https://doi.org/10.9778/cmajo.20210239

Hallinan, C. M., Gunn, J. M., & Bonomo, Y. A. (2021). Implementation of medicinal cannabis in Australia: Innovation or upheaval? Perspectives from physicians as key informants, a qualitative analysis. *British Medical Journal Open, 11*(10), e054044. https://doi.org/10.1136/bmjopen-2021-054044

Hordowicz, M., Jarosz, J., Czaplińska, M., Leonhard, A., & Klimkiewicz, A. (2021). Polish physicians' perspectives on medical cannabis policy and educational needs: Results of an online survey. *Journal of Clinical Medicine, 10*(19), 4545. https://doi.org/10.3390/jcm10194545

Manoharan, R., Kemper, J., & Young, J. (2022). Exploring the medical cannabis prescribing behaviours of New Zealand physicians. *Drug and Alcohol Review, 41*(6), 1355–1366. https://doi.org/10.1111/dar.13476

Mansell, H., Zaslawski, Z., Kelly, L. E., Lougheed, T., Brace, T., & Alcorn, J. (2022). Medical cannabis in schools: A qualitative study on the experiences of clinicians. *Paediatrics & Child Health, 28*(2), 113–118. https://doi.org/10.1093/pch/pxac110

Ng, J. Y., Gilotra, K., Usman, S., Chang, Y., & Busse, J. W. (2021). Attitudes toward medical cannabis among family physicians practising in Ontario, Canada: A qualitative research study. *CMAJ Open, 9*(2), E342–E348. https://doi.org/10.9778/cmajo.20200187

Ng, J. Y., Quach, H., Phillips, M. R., & Busse, J. W. (2022). Surveying Canadian pain physicians' attitudes and beliefs regarding medical cannabis for chronic noncancer pain: A qualitative study. *Journal of Pain Research, 15*, 3899–3910. https://doi.org/10.2147/JPR.S382589

Orjuela-Rojas, J. M., García Orjuela, X., & Ocampo Serna, S. (2021). Medicinal cannabis: Knowledge, beliefs, and attitudes of Colombian psychiatrists. *Journal of Cannabis Research, 3*(1), 26. https://doi.org/10.1186/s42238-021-00083-z

Reece, S. M., Holle, L., & Mukherjee, K. (2021). Survey of pharmacists' knowledge of Connecticut's medical cannabis program. *Cannabis and Cannabinoid Research, 6*(1), 66–73. https://doi.org/10.1089/can.2019.0013

Rønne, S. T., Rosenaek, F., Pedersen, L. B., Waldorff, F. B., Nielsen, J. B., Riisgaard, H., & Søndergaard, J. (2021). Physicians' experiences, attitudes, and beliefs towards medical cannabis: A systematic literature review. *BMC Family Practice, 22*(1), 212. https://doi.org/10.1186/s12875-021-01559-w

Rosenbaek, F., Riisgaard, H., Nielsen, J. B., Wehberg, S., Waldorff, F. B., Pedersen, L. B., & Søndergaard, J. (2023). GPs' prescription patterns, experience, and attitudes towards medicinal cannabis-a nationwide survey at the early stage of the Danish test scheme. *BMC Primary Care, 24*(1), 17. https://doi.org/10.1186/s12875-023-01971-4

Sabmeethavorn, Q., Bonomo, Y. A., & Hallinan, C. M. (2022). Pharmacists' perceptions and experiences of medicinal cannabis dispensing: A narrative review with a systematic approach. *The International Journal of Pharmacy Practice, 30*(3), 204–214. https://doi.org/10.1093/ijpp/riac005

Chapter 4
Future Research Directions and Closing Remarks

Abstract This chapter begins with a section that explains the existing gaps in our knowledge about the therapeutic benefits that medical/medicinal cannabis can give patients. It then explains the gaps in our understanding about the experiences of healthcare professionals prescribing medical/medicinal cannabis to their patients. This chapter concludes with a summary of this book.

Keywords Control groups · Member checking · Missing data · Non-representative samples · Small sample sizes

4.1 Medical/Medicinal Cannabis for Disabilities and Medical and Psychological Conditions

4.1.1 No Control Groups

Within five studies, it was impossible to accurately determine the therapeutic benefits and side effects of cannabis on participants because there was no control group (Bapir et al., 2023; Ergisi et al., 2022; Erridge et al., 2022; Nacasch et al., 2023; Pillai et al., 2022). To ensure that the benefits and dangers of cannabis are accurately measured, studies in future should contain a control group. However, researchers need to carefully consider the ethics of withholding a substance from participants in a control group that might give them therapeutic benefits.

4.1.2 Previous Usage of Medical/Medicinal Cannabis Products

Within four studies, participants had already been consuming cannabis before the study started (Ittiphakorn et al., 2023; Krediet et al., 2020; Mangoo et al., 2022; Rifkin-Zybute et al., 2023). For example, in Ittiphakorn et al.'s (2023) study most

G. Bennett, *A Scoping Review of Clinical Studies About the Therapeutic Benefits of Medical Cannabis*, https://doi.org/10.1007/978-981-97-7941-3_4

participants (80.88%) were already taking cannabis before staring the study. Pre-usage of cannabis could have skewed the results because it is possible that the results reported were in favour of those who had positive experiences of cannabis and those who had a negative experience of cannabis would have been reluctant to enrol in the study.

4.1.3 Missing Data

In several studies, details from the participants that could have improved the understanding of the results were not collected. For example, Sachedina et al. (2022) did not collect details from participants about their pharmaceutical and/or non-pharmaceutical therapy at the beginning of their study. Such treatment programmes might have had an impact on the effectiveness of cannabis treatment. To ensure that the therapeutic potential of cannabis is accurately measured, participants not using other therapies should be recruited into studies about the therapeutic benefits of medical/medicinal cannabis.

4.1.4 Small Sample Size

Within several studies, the sample size was too small for any conclusions to be generalised to the population (Krediet et al., 2020). To ensure that the results of the study can be generalised to the entire population, it is important that sample sizes are increased.

4.1.5 Non-representative Sample

Within six studies, the authors explained that due to various reasons their samples contained a homogeneous group of participants, which limited the ability of the findings to be generalised to the population. For example, for Ergisi et al.'s (2022), Erridge et al.'s (2023), Bapir et al.'s (2023), Ittiphakorn et al.'s (2023), and Sachedina et al.'s (2022) studies, all participants were recruited from the same private clinic. Similarly, 85% of participants in Rifkin-Zybutz et al. (2023) study had previously consumed or were consuming non-pharmaceutical grade cannabis products when they began the study. To ensure that the samples are more representative of the population, the size of the sample should be increased and participants should be recruited from multiple locations.

4.1.6 Subjectivity of Patient-Reported Outcome Measures (PROMs)

Within Suraev et al. (2023) and Sznitman et al. (2022), the results were based on the self-reported recollections of participants. Such self-reported accounts can undermine the accurate evaluation of the efficacy and side effects of medical/medicinal cannabis. While self-reported experiences are important, they should be accompanied with objective measurements of the effectiveness and drawbacks of medical/medicinal cannabis.

4.2 Healthcare Professionals Prescribing Medical/Medicinal Cannabis

4.2.1 Small Sample Size and Non-representative Sample

Within five studies, the authors explained that the study's results were based on small sample sizes (Adler et al., 2022; Alharbi et al., 2023; Bawa et al., 2023; Manoharan et al., 2022; Rosenbæk et al., 2023). For example, the response rate in Rosenbæk et al.'s (2023) study was 38.4%. In another example, Adler et al. (2022) explained that their response rate was 23.6%. Due to these small response rates, it is difficult to create generalisations from the data collected. Similarly, Adler et al. also explained that due to the voluntary nature of their study physicians with staunch opinions, whether they be in favour or against medical cannabis, may have been more inclined to respond. Their inclination to participate may have created selection bias. To mitigate the prospect of selection bias and to improve the generalisability of the findings, undertaking studies with larger sample sizes would be prudent.

4.2.2 Professionals Recruited from a Single Location

The authors within three studies claimed that they had sourced participants from a single location (Bui et al., 2023; Mansell et al., 2022; Orjuela-Rojas et al., 2021). For example, Orjuela-Rojas et al. (2021) explained that most psychiatrists surveyed for their study were recruited from Cundinamarca, particularly in Bogotá, the capital. In future, researchers should recruit participants from other locations so that the generalisability of the results can occur.

4.2.3 No Member Checking

Gunning et al. (2022) and Ng et al. (2021) explained that the interview transcripts were not returned to the participants so that they could check the accuracy of the answers that they provided. To ensure that the responses collected from participants are accurate, in the future it would be prudent for researchers to give the data collected back to the participants for them to verify.

4.3 Concluding Comments

This book had two main objectives. First, to present an overview to the reader about the main findings in the literature about the benefits and drawbacks of using medical/medicinal cannabis to treat disabilities, or medical or psychological conditions. Second, to describe the documented experiences and insights in the literature from medical professionals, patients, and pharmacists about using or prescribing medical/medicinal cannabis.

The literature reported in Chapter two revealed that medical/medicinal cannabis had therapeutic benefits for people with various disabilities and diseases. It was reported that it helped people with attention-deficit hyperactivity disorder manage their anxiety and sleeping difficulties (Ittiphakorn et al., 2023). Additionally, for people with multiple sclerosis cannabis was discovered to potentially decrease their chronic pain, muscle spasticity, and sleep disturbances (Rainka et al., 2023). Despite these discoveries, within multiple studies there was a dominant view that more research should be undertaken to confirm published findings (Efron & Taylor, 2023; Sznitman et al., 2022).

Despite its benefits, medicinal/medical cannabis can have side effects for people with disabilities and/or medical conditions and/or psychological conditions. For example, Fletcher et al. (2022) reported that participants in their sample reported experiencing somnolence (n = 19/251, 7.6%), decreased appetite (n = 13/251, 5.2%), and gastrointestinal symptoms (n = 12/251, 4.8%). Due to the prospect of side effects, more research needs to be conducted to ensure that correct dosages of medicinal/medical cannabis are given to patients. Additionally, more research needs to be conducted to ensure that the benefits of medicinal/medical cannabis outweigh the associated risks.

The views and experiences of medical professionals prescribing, or intending to prescribe, medical/medicinal cannabis was explored in the previous chapter. The current literature shows that although some medical professionals are receptive to prescribing medical/medicinal cannabis to their patients, they are unsure about the legislative consequences (Orjuela-Rojas et al., 2021). Similarly, in Bawa et al.'s (2023) study 61.3% of participants expressed that they had a lack of training/resources regarding prescribing medical/medicinal cannabis. Due to their lack of pharmacological, legislative, and regulatory knowledge about prescribing medical/medicinal cannabis, it is advised that more training should be provided to pharmacists.

This book contains a summary of the literature about people using medical/medicinal cannabis and medical professionals prescribing or dispensing this medication to patients. Despite the summarised views, the results in the studies are often based on small and homogeneous sample and on the subjective self-reported recollections of participants. In future, researchers should take these limitations into consideration when they are designing their studies. For example, to mitigate results being based on a homogenous sample of participants, researchers should ensure that they have recruited participants from a broader geographical area and from public and private clinics and institutions.

References

Adler, L., Zacay, G., Schonmann, Y., Azuri, J., Yehoshua, I., Vinker, S., Shani, M., Heymann, A. D., & Hoffman, R. (2022). Primary care physicians' attitudes and knowledge regarding medical cannabis and willingness to prescribe it: The Israeli experience. *Family Practice, 39*(1), 59–64. https://doi.org/10.1093/fampra/cmab108

Alharbi, F. F., Alqahtani, T. M., Alzamil, A. M., Alharbi, N. H., & Masud, N. (2023). Knowledge, perception, and beliefs of Saudi physicians at King Abdulaziz Medical City, Riyadh related to medical cannabis: Literature review and a cross-sectional survey. *Journal of Family Medicine and Primary Care, 12*(3), 536–544. https://doi.org/10.4103/jfmpc.jfmpc_1856_22

Bapir, L., Erridge, S., Nicholas, M., Pillai, M., Dalavaye, N., Holvey, C., Coomber, R., Hoare, J., Khan, S., Weatherall, M. W., Rucker, J. J., Platt, M., & Sodergren, M. H. (2023). Comparing the effects of medical cannabis for chronic pain patients with and without co-morbid anxiety: A cohort study. *Expert Review of Neurotherapeutics, 23*(3), 281–295. https://doi.org/10.1080/14737175.2023.2181696

Bawa, Z., Saini, B., McCartney, D., Bedoya-Pérez, M., McLachlan, A. J., & McGregor, I. S. (2023). A cross-sectional survey exploring the knowledge, experiences and attitudes of Australian pharmacists toward medicinal cannabis. *International Journal of Clinical Pharmacy, 45*(2), 375–386. https://doi.org/10.1007/s11096-022-01519-z

Bui, K., Worster, B., Ryan, J., Pant, S., & Kelly, E. L. (2023). Physicians' perspectives on their training for and role within Pennsylvania's medical cannabis program. *Journal of the American Board of Family Medicine, 36*(4), 670–681. https://doi.org/10.3122/jabfm.2022.220304R1

Efron, D., & Taylor, K. (2023). Medicinal cannabis for paediatric developmental, behavioural and mental health disorders. *International Journal of Environmental Research and Public Health, 20*(8), 5430. https://doi.org/10.3390/ijerph20085430

Ergisi, M., Erridge, S., Harris, M., Kawka, M., Nimalan, D., Salazar, O., Loupasaki, K., Ali, R., Holvey, C., Coomber, R., Platt, M., Rucker, J. J., & Sodergren, M. H. (2022). UK medical cannabis registry: An analysis of clinical outcomes of medicinal cannabis therapy for generalized anxiety disorder. *Expert Review of Clinical Pharmacology, 15*(4), 487–495. https://doi.org/10.1080/17512433.2022.2020640

Erridge, S., Holvey, C., Coomber, R., Hoare, J., Khan, S., Platt, M. W., Rucker, J. J., Weatherall, M. W., Beri, S., & Sodergren, M. H. (2023). Clinical outcome data of children treated with cannabis-based medicinal products for treatment resistant epilepsy-analysis from the UK medical cannabis registry. *Neuropediatrics, 54*(3), 174–181. https://doi.org/10.1055/a-2002-2119

Erridge, S., Kerr-Gaffney, J., Holvey, C., Coomber, R., Barros, D. A. R., Bhoskar, U., Mwimba, G., Praveen, K., Symeon, C., Sachdeva-Mohan, S., Sodergren, M. H., & Rucker, J. J. (2022). Clinical outcome analysis of patients with autism spectrum disorder: Analysis from the UK medical cannabis registry. *Therapeutic Advances in Psychopharmacology, 12*, 20451253221116240. https://doi.org/10.1177/20451253221116240

Fletcher, S., Pawliuk, C., Ip, A., Huh, L., Rassekh, S. R., Oberlander, T. F., & Siden, H. (2022). Medicinal cannabis in children and adolescents with autism spectrum disorder: A scoping review. *Child: Care, Health and Development, 48*(1), 33–44. https://doi.org/10.1111/cch.12909

Gunning, M., Rotenberg, A. D., Kelly, L. E., Crooks, B., Oberoi, S., Rapoport, A. L., Rassekh, S. R., & Illes, J. (2022). Clinician views on and ethics priorities for authorizing medical cannabis in the care of children and youth in Canada: A qualitative study. *CMAJ Open, 10*(1), E196–E202. https://doi.org/10.9778/cmajo.20210239

Ittiphakorn, P., Erridge, S., Holvey, C., Coomber, R., Rucker, J. J., & Sodergren, M. H. (2023). UK medical cannabis registry: An analysis of clinical outcomes of medicinal cannabis therapy for attention-deficit/hyperactivity disorder. *Neuropsychopharmacology Reports, 43*(4), 596–606. https://doi.org/10.1002/npr2.12400

Krediet, E., Janssen, D. G., Heerdink, E. R., Egberts, T. C., & Vermetten, E. (2020). Experiences with medical cannabis in the treatment of veterans with PTSD: Results from a focus group discussion. *European Neuropsychopharmacology: The Journal of the European College of Neuropsychopharmacology, 36*, 244–254. https://doi.org/10.1016/j.euroneuro.2020.04.009

Mangoo, S., Erridge, S., Holvey, C., Coomber, R., Barros, D. A. R., Bhoskar, U., Mwimba, G., Praveen, K., Symeon, C., Sachdeva-Mohan, S., Rucker, J. J., & Sodergren, M. H. (2022). Assessment of clinical outcomes of medicinal cannabis therapy for depression: Analysis from the UK medical cannabis registry. *Expert Review of Neurotherapeutics, 22*(11–12), 995–1008. https://doi.org/10.1080/14737175.2022.2161894

Manoharan, R., Kemper, J., & Young, J. (2022). Exploring the medical cannabis prescribing behaviours of New Zealand physicians. *Drug and Alcohol Review, 41*(6), 1355–1366. https://doi.org/10.1111/dar.13476

Mansell, H., Zaslawski, Z., Kelly, L. E., Lougheed, T., Brace, T., & Alcorn, J. (2022). Medical cannabis in schools: A qualitative study on the experiences of clinicians. *Paediatrics & Child Health, 28*(2), 113–118. https://doi.org/10.1093/pch/pxac110

Nacasch, N., Avni, C., & Toren, P. (2023). Medical cannabis for treatment-resistant combat PTSD. *Frontiers in Psychiatry, 13*, 1014630. https://doi.org/10.3389/fpsyt.2022.1014630

Ng, J. Y., Gilotra, K., Usman, S., Chang, Y., & Busse, J. W. (2021). Attitudes toward medical cannabis among family physicians practising in Ontario, Canada: A qualitative research study. *CMAJ Open, 9*(2), E342–E348. https://doi.org/10.9778/cmajo.20200187

Orjuela-Rojas, J. M., García Orjuela, X., & Ocampo Serna, S. (2021). Medicinal cannabis: Knowledge, beliefs, and attitudes of Colombian psychiatrists. *Journal of Cannabis Research, 3*(1), 26. https://doi.org/10.1186/s42238-021-00083-z

Pillai, M., Erridge, S., Bapir, L., Nicholas, M., Dalavaye, N., Holvey, C., Coomber, R., Barros, D., Bhoskar, U., Mwimba, G., Praveen, K., Symeon, C., Sachdeva-Mohan, S., Rucker, J. J., & Sodergren, M. H. (2022). Assessment of clinical outcomes in patients with post-traumatic stress disorder: Analysis from the UK medical cannabis registry. *Expert Review of Neurotherapeutics, 22*(11–12), 1009–1018. https://doi.org/10.1080/14737175.2022.2155139

Rainka, M. M., Aladeen, T. S., Mattle, A. G., Lewandowski, E., Vanini, D., McCormack, K., & Mechtler, L. (2023). Multiple sclerosis and use of medical cannabis: A retrospective review of a neurology outpatient population. *International Journal of MS Care, 25*(3), 111–117. https://doi.org/10.7224/1537-2073.2022-006

Rifkin-Zybutz, R., Erridge, S., Holvey, C., Coomber, R., Gaffney, J., Lawn, W., Barros, D., Bhoskar, U., Mwimba, G., Praveen, K., Symeon, C., Sachdeva-Mohan, S., Rucker, J. J., & Sodergren, M. H. (2023). Clinical outcome data of anxiety patients treated with cannabis-based medicinal products in the United Kingdom: A cohort study from the UK medical cannabis registry. *Psychopharmacology (Berl), 240*(8), 1735–1745. https://doi.org/10.1007/s00213-023-06399-3

Rosenbæk, F., Riisgaard, H., Nielsen, J. B., Wehberg, S., Waldorff, F. B., Pedersen, L. B., & Søndergaard, J. (2023). GPs' prescription patterns, experience, and attitudes towards medicinal cannabis-a nationwide survey at the early stage of the Danish test scheme. *BMC Primary Care, 24*(1), 17. https://doi.org/10.1186/s12875-023-01971-4

Sachedina, F., Chan, C., Damji, R. S., & de Sanctis, O. J. (2022). Medical cannabis use in Canada and its impact on anxiety and depression: A retrospective study. *Psychiatry Research, 313*, 114573. https://doi.org/10.1016/j.psychres.2022.114573

Suraev, A., Mills, L., Abelev, S. V., Arkell, T. R., Lintzeris, N., & McGregor, I. S. (2023). Medical cannabis use patterns for sleep disorders in Australia: Results of the cross-sectional CAMS-20 survey. *Nature and Science of Sleep, 15*, 245–255. https://doi.org/10.2147/NSS.S390583

Sznitman, S. R., Meiri, D., Amit, B. H., Rosenberg, D., & Greene, T. (2022). Posttraumatic stress disorder, sleep and medical cannabis treatment: A daily diary study. *Journal of Anxiety Disorders, 92*, 102632. https://doi.org/10.1016/j.janxdis.2022.102632

Appendix A
Comparison of Current Licenced and Unlicenced Medicinal Cannabis Products Available in the United Kingdom

Name	Form	Composition	Licenced indication	Possible indication for people with intellectual disabilities
Epidyolex (Electronic medicines compendium, 2022)	Liquid	CBD 100 mg/ml	Seizures in children (aged two or older) with two rare forms of epilepsy, Lennox–Gastaut syndrome and Dravet syndrome, in conjunction with clobazam, and as adjunctive therapy of seizures associated with tuberous sclerosis complex	For persons with ID with co-occurring epilepsy, with uncontrolled seizures contributing to the challenging behaviour (e.g. during peri-ictal period), as well as severe anxiety and challenging behaviour
Sativex (Electronic Medicines Compendium, 2022)	Oromucosal spray	Each ml contains: 27 mg THC and 25 mg CBD	Multiple sclerosis associated spasticity unresponsive to other treatments	This medication has been found to be effective to treat tic disorder (Koppel, 2015). Tics are another common co-occurring condition with neurodevelopmental conditions
Nabilone (Electronic Medicines Compendium, 2021)	Capsule	Synthetic cannabinoid (mimics effect of THC)	Chemotherapy-induced nausea and vomiting unresponsive to conventional anti-emetics	No clear indication

(continued)

G. Bennett, *A Scoping Review of Clinical Studies About the Therapeutic Benefits of Medical Cannabis*, https://doi.org/10.1007/978-981-97-7941-3

(continued)

Name	Form	Composition	Licenced indication	Possible indication for people with intellectual disabilities
CBD: THC products	Drops (oil) or inhaled (dried flower)	CBD and THC titrated up as per dosing protocol of the prescribing clinic	No current licensed indications. These forms are prescribed in private practice (off-label and off-licenced use)	There is real-world observational data and emerging evidence suggesting improvements in several mental health conditions associated with challenging behaviour including anxiety, post-traumatic stress disorder (PTSD), autism and ADHD
Over the counter and internet CBD products (Chesney et al., 2020)	Drops (oil), gummies, capsules, spray	Often marketed as 'pure CBD' but could contain low amounts of CBD or some THC, as products are not regulated	No current licenced indications. Health stores claim that CBD products have a range of indications including pain relief, anxiety insomnia, PTSD related symptoms, depression and lowering blood pressure	Not advisable given the lack of control over the dosing and lack of medical guidance

Source Korb et al. (2023, p. 1203)

References

Chesney, E., McGuire, P., Freeman, T. P., Strang, J., & Englund, A. (2020). Lack of evidence for the effectiveness or safety of over-the-counter cannabidiol products. *Therapeutic Advances in Psychopharmacology*, *10*, 2045125320954992. https://doi.org/10.1177/2045125320954992

Electronic Medicines Compendium. (2021). *Nabilone 1 mg Capsule.* https://www.medicines.org.uk/emc/product/12767/smpc#gref

Electronic Medicines Compendium. (2022). *Epidyolex 100 mg/ml oral solution.* https://www.medicines.org.uk/emc/product/10781#gref

Koppel, B. S. (2015). Cannabis in the Treatment of Dystonia, Dyskinesias, and Tics. *Neurotherapeutics: The Journal of the American Society for Experimental NeuroTherapeutics*, *12*(4), 788–792. https://doi.org/10.1007/s13311-015-0376-4

Korb, L., Tromans, S., Perera, B., Khan, N., Burrows, L., Laugharne, R., Hassiotis, A., Allgar, V., Efron, D., Maidment, I., & Shankar, R. (2023). The potential for medicinal cannabis to help manage challenging behaviour in people with intellectual disability: A perspective review. *Journal of Psychopharmacology (Oxford, England)*, *37*(12), 1201–1208. https://doi.org/10.1177/02698811231209192

Appendix B
Dataset

PubMed ID	First author surname	Article title	DOI number	Citation included in the study (yes/no)
38155535	Murphy	A cohort study comparing the effects of medical cannabis for anxiety patients with and without comorbid sleep disturbance	https://doi.org/10.1002/npr2.12407	Yes
38126843	Lupke	Impacts of medicinal cannabis on an early psychosis service	https://doi.org/10.1177/10398562231222818	No
38100798	Hong	Legal and regulatory aspects of medical cannabis in the United States	https://doi.org/10.1213/ANE.0000000000006301	No
38094100	Strand	Medical cannabis: a review from the American Society of pain and neuroscience	https://doi.org/10.2147/JPR.S425862	No
38071933	Anderson	Impact of non-medical cannabis legalization with market restrictions on health service use and incident cases of psychotic disorder in Ontario, Canada	https://doi.org/10.1016/j.drugpo.2023.104285	No
38058251	Ittiphakorn	UK medical cannabis registry: an analysis of clinical outcomes of medicinal cannabis therapy for attention-deficit/hyperactivity disorder	https://doi.org/10.1002/npr2.12400	Yes
38057993	Erridge	An observational study of clinical outcome measures in patients treated with cannabis-based medicinal products on the UK medical cannabis registry	https://doi.org/10.1002/npr2.12403	No

(continued)

G. Bennett, *A Scoping Review of Clinical Studies About the Therapeutic Benefits of Medical Cannabis*, https://doi.org/10.1007/978-981-97-7941-3

(continued)

PubMed ID	First author surname	Article title	DOI number	Citation included in the study (yes/no)
38041708	Lee	Medical cannabis and its efficacy/effectiveness for the treatment of low-back pain: a systematic review	https://doi.org/10.1007/s11916-023-01189-0	No
38027232	Dassieu	Experiences and perceptions of medical cannabis among people living with chronic pain and community pharmacists: a qualitative study in Canada	https://doi.org/10.1080/24740527.2023.2258537	Yes
38026946	Baratta	Editorial: medicinal Cannabis: evolution of therapeutic use, future approaches and other implications, volume II	https://doi.org/10.3389/fphar.2023.1322404	No
38015317	Hidding	Therapeutic use of medical Cannabis in neurological diseases: a clinical update	https://doi.org/10.1007/s00702-023-02719-1	No
37973200	Sharon	Medical cannabis for refractory cancer-related pain in a specialised clinical service: a cross-sectional study	https://doi.org/10.1136/spcare-2023-004421	No
37963569	Morano	Medicinal cannabis: extended stability of cannabis extracts produced using a new ethanol-based extraction method	https://doi.org/10.1055/a-2189-8155	No
37952701	Dewidar	Operationalizing the GRADE-equity criterion to inform guideline recommendations: application to a medical cannabis guideline	https://doi.org/10.1016/j.jclinepi.2023.10.001	No
37945917	Arkell	A semi-naturalistic, open-label trial examining the effect of prescribed medical cannabis on neurocognitive performance	https://doi.org/10.1007/s40263-023-01046-z	No
37941019	Jylkkä	The holistic effects of medical cannabis compared to opioids on pain experience in Finnish patients with chronic pain	https://doi.org/10.1186/s42238-023-00207-7	No
37937428	Korb	The potential for medicinal cannabis to help manage challenging behaviour in people with intellectual disability: a perspective review	https://doi.org/10.1177/02698811231209192	Yes
37923347	Bicket	Association of cannabis use with patient-reported pain measures among adults with chronic pain in US states with medical cannabis programs	https://doi.org/10.1136/rapm-2023-104833	No
37920683	Valikhanova	Medical cannabis use among Canadian veterans and non-veterans: a national survey	https://doi.org/10.1089/imr.2023.0022	No

(continued)

(continued)

PubMed ID	First author surname	Article title	DOI number	Citation included in the study (yes/no)
37900896	Kluwe	Medical cannabis alleviates chronic neuropathic pain effectively and sustainably without severe adverse effect: a retrospective study on 99 cases	https://doi.org/10.1159/000531667	No
37893071	Abuhasira	Medical Cannabis is not associated with a decrease in activities of daily living in older adults	https://doi.org/10.3390/biomedicines11102697	No
37886802	Wootten	The effect of non-medical cannabis retailer proximity on use of mental health services for psychotic disorders in Ontario, Canada	https://doi.org/10.1177/00207640231206053	No
37885234	Ney	Challenges and considerations for treating PTSD with medicinal cannabis: the Australian clinician's perspective	https://doi.org/10.1080/17512433.2023.2276309	No
37884682	Wardill	Supporting gut health with medicinal cannabis in people with advanced cancer: potential benefits and challenges	https://doi.org/10.1038/s41416-023-02466-w	No
37884027	Alexander	Medical cannabis legalization: no contribution to rising stimulant rates in the USA	https://doi.org/10.1055/a-2152-7757	No
37873024	Poisblaud	Perceptions and preoccupations of patients and physicians regarding use of medical cannabis as an intervention against chronic musculoskeletal pain: results from a qualitative study	https://doi.org/10.2147/JPR.S413450	No
37855429	Sinclair	"A glimmer of hope"—perceptions, barriers, and drivers for medicinal cannabis use amongst Australian and New Zealand people with endometriosis	https://doi.org/10.1530/RAF-23-0049	No
37843897	Lunn	Letter to the editor: medical cannabis in Canada: the need for insurance coverage expansion	https://doi.org/10.1089/can.2023.0120	No
37837446	Gurgenci	Exploring potential anti-inflammatory effects of medicinal cannabis	https://doi.org/10.1007/s00520-023-08069-8	No

(continued)

(continued)

PubMed ID	First author surname	Article title	DOI number	Citation included in the study (yes/no)
37819556	Grant	Knowledge and attitudes towards medicinal cannabis and complementary and integrative medicine (CIM): a survey of healthcare professionals working in a cancer hospital in Australia	https://doi.org/10.1007/s00520-023-08080-z	No
37813082	Graham	A provisional evaluation of Australia's medical cannabis program	https://doi.org/10.1016/j.drugpo.2023	No
37767954	Fehr	Stigma-related barriers to medical cannabis as harm reduction for substance use disorder: obstacles and opportunities for improvement	https://doi.org/10.1111/inm.13231	No
37748856	Lee	Drug dependence epidemiology in palliative care medicinal cannabis trials	https://doi.org/10.1136/spcare-2023-004583	No
37732650	Eloise	Medical cannabis	https://doi.org/10.1097/01.NAJ.0000979020.71276.1b	No
37719209	Ahmed	Enhanced production of select phytocannabinoids in medical cannabis cultivars using microbial consortia	https://doi.org/10.3389/fpls.2023.1219836	No
37701550	Storey	Views on and experiences with medicinal cannabis among Canadian veterans who live with pain: a qualitative study	https://doi.org/10.1080/24740527.2023.2232838	No
37677985	Balneaves	Baccalaureate nursing students' knowledge, attitudes, educational needs, and use of medical and non-medical cannabis at five institutions in Manitoba, Canada: a cross-sectional analysis	https://doi.org/10.1016/j.nedt.2023.105955	No
37674243	Arkell	Driving-related behaviors, attitudes, and perceptions among Australian medical cannabis users: results from the CAMS 20 survey	https://doi.org/10.1186/s42238-023-00202-y	No
37672515	Tait	Health-related quality of life in patients accessing medicinal cannabis in Australia: the QUEST initiative results of a 3-month follow-up observational study	https://doi.org/10.1371/journal.pone.0290549	No

(continued)

(continued)

PubMed ID	First author surname	Article title	DOI number	Citation included in the study (yes/no)
37632419		Medicinal cannabis and implications for workplace health and safety: scoping review of systematic reviews	https://doi.org/10.1177/21650799231172722	No
37626819	Christensen	Decoding the postulated entourage effect of medicinal cannabis: what it is and what it isn't	https://doi.org/10.3390/biomedicines11082323	No
37608004	Quillet	A machine learning approach for understanding the metabolomics response of children with autism spectrum disorder to medical cannabis treatment	https://doi.org/10.1038/s41598-023-40073-0	No
37581814	Tsampoula	Quality of life in patients receiving medical cannabis	https://doi.org/10.1007/978-3-031-31986-0_39	No
37572391	Cook	Medical cannabis laws lower individual market health insurance premiums	https://doi.org/10.1016/j.drugpo.2023.104143	No
37562842	Bui	Physicians' perspectives on their training for and role within Pennsylvania's medical cannabis program	https://doi.org/10.3122/jabfm.2022.220304R1	Yes
37546945	Syed	International perspective on physician knowledge, attitude and practices related to medical cannabis	https://doi.org/10.1101/2023.07.26.23293157	No
37538850	Lyu	Medical cannabis received by patients according to qualifying condition in a US state cannabis program: product choice, dosing, and age-related trends	https://doi.org/10.1016/j.curtheres.2023.100709	No
37520218	Sokratous	Attitudes, beliefs, and knowledge regarding medical cannabis among healthcare students in the Republic of Cyprus: a cross-sectional descriptive correlational study	https://doi.org/10.3389/fpsyt.2023.1196915	No
37519131	Boehnke	Medicinal cannabis use for rheumatic conditions in the US versus Canada: rationale for use and patient-health care provider interactions	https://doi.org/10.1002/acr2.11592	No
37514290	Morad	Response of medical cannabis to magnesium (Mg) supply at the vegetative growth phase	https://doi.org/10.3390/plants12142676	No

(continued)

(continued)

PubMed ID	First author surname	Article title	DOI number	Citation included in the study (yes/no)
37500826	Myran	Association between non-medical cannabis legalization and emergency department visits for cannabis-induced psychosis	https://doi.org/10.1038/s41380-023-02185-x	No
37484054	Gebru	"That's pot culture right there": purchasing behaviors of people who use cannabis without a medical cannabis card	https://doi.org/10.26828/cannabis/2023/000168	No
37484052	McMahon	Perceived effectiveness of medical cannabis among adults with chronic pain: findings from interview data in a three-month pilot study	https://doi.org/10.26828/cannabis/2023/000149	No
37467000	Harris	Medical cannabis did not reduce pain prescriptions, procedures	https://doi.org/10.1001/jama.2023.12554	No
37456642	Anis	A single-center real-life study on the use of medical cannabis in patients with dystonia	https://doi.org/10.3389/fneur.2023.1218300	No
37434242	Alvarez	Conflicting forces in the implementation of medicinal cannabis regulation in Uruguay	https://doi.org/10.1186/s42238-023-00189-6	No
37414508	Colby	Medical cannabis program sustainability in the era of recreational cannabis	https://doi.org/10.1016/j.clinthera.2023.01.017	No
37414507	McNabb	Self-reported medicinal cannabis use as an alternative to prescription and over-the-counter medication use among US military veterans	https://doi.org/10.1016/j.clinthera.2023.04.003	No
37414503	Graham	Medicinal cannabis guidance and resources for health professionals to inform clinical decision making	https://doi.org/10.1016/j.clinthera.2023.03.007	No
37399549	McGinty	Effects of U.S. state medical cannabis laws on treatment of chronic noncancer pain	https://doi.org/10.7326/M23-0053	No
37390030	Withanarachchie	Barriers and facilitators to prescribing medicinal cannabis in New Zealand	https://doi.org/10.1071/HC22122	No
37385763	Rashid	Yonder: pre-operative anxiety, breast cancer screening, patient decision aids, and medicinal cannabis	https://doi.org/10.3399/bjgp23X733353	No

(continued)

(continued)

PubMed ID	First author surname	Article title	DOI number	Citation included in the study (yes/no)
37384372	O'Neill	Evaluating the supporting evidence of medical cannabis claims made on clinic websites: cross-sectional study	https://doi.org/10.2196/45550	No
37346297	Cairns	Medicinal cannabis for psychiatry-related conditions: an overview of current Australian prescribing	https://doi.org/10.3389/fphar.2023.1142680	No
37345762	Johnson	Increasing patient access to medical cannabis requires federal legislation	https://doi.org/10.1097/01.NAJ.0000944852.53378.0f	No
37338932	McQuoid	Outdoor medical cannabis advertising in Oklahoma: examining regulatory compliance and social meanings in billboard content	https://doi.org/10.1080/10826084.2023.2223299	No
37314478	Rifkin-Zybutz	Clinical outcome data of anxiety patients treated with cannabis-based medicinal products in the United Kingdom: a cohort study from the UK medical cannabis registry	https://doi.org/10.1007/s00213-023-06399-3	Yes
37299195	Favero	Alternative rooting methods for medicinal cannabis cultivation in denmark-preliminary results	https://doi.org/10.3390/plants12112216	No
37296470	Minhas	Naturalistic examination of the anxiolytic effects of medical cannabis and associated gender and age differences in a Canadian cohort	https://doi.org/10.1186/s42238-023-00192-x	No
37292156	Stith	Understanding feeling "high" and its role in medical cannabis patient outcomes	https://doi.org/10.3389/fphar.2023.1135453	No
37287727	Steuart	State Variation in U.S. medical cannabis limits, restrictions, and therapeutic cannabis dosing	https://doi.org/10.26828/cannabis/2023.01.001	No
37285183	Tanco	Analysis of dispensing and utilization patterns of medical cannabis products in state licensed cannabis dispensaries	https://doi.org/10.1089/jpm.2023.0075	No
37283486	Häuser	Cannabis-based medicines and medical cannabis for adults with cancer pain	https://doi.org/10.1002/14651858.CD014915.pub2	No
37283094	Smith	Quality of life beyond measure: advanced cancer patients, wellbeing and medicinal cannabis	https://doi.org/10.1111/1467-9566.13684	No

(continued)

(continued)

PubMed ID	First author surname	Article title	DOI number	Citation included in the study (yes/no)
37261066	Sajdeya	Protocol of a combined cohort and cross-sectional study of persons receiving medical cannabis in Florida, USA: the medical marijuana and me (M(3)) study	https://doi.org/10.1159/000530052	No
37257363	Syed	Impact of personal beliefs about medical cannabis on physician recommendation practices: results of an international survey	https://doi.org/10.1016/j.ajp.2023.103634	No
37250194	Rainka	Multiple sclerosis and use of medical cannabis: a retrospective review of a neurology outpatient population	https://doi.org/10.7224/1537-2073.2022-006	Yes
37246101	Barré	French general practitioners and medical cannabis: a need for training	https://doi.org/10.1016/j.encep.2023.04.006	No
37244526	Cohen	Use of medical cannabis by patients with cancer: attitudes, knowledge, and practice	https://doi.org/10.1016/j.jpainsymman.2023.05.010	No
37243499	Ne'eman-Haviv	Public perceptions of medical cannabis diversion: a legal and moral dilemma	https://doi.org/10.1177/13591053231173590	No
37214833	Stains	Is medical cannabis evidence-based medicine? Concerns based on qualifying conditions and the national academy of sciences report	https://doi.org/10.1101/2023.05.01.23289286	No
37214578	Fiore	Medicinal cannabis products for the treatment of acute pain	https://doi.org/10.12998/wjcc.v11.i12.2670	No
37213732	Clobes	Demographic factors that impact attitudes toward medical cannabis	https://doi.org/10.1016/j.pecinn.2022.100085	No
37211456	Goldberg	Long-term safety of medical cannabis in Parkinson's disease: a retrospective case–control study	https://doi.org/10.1016/j.parkreldis.2023.105406	Yes—article was behind a paywall and could not be accessed
37207711	Hernandez	Changes in Arkansans' attitudes toward pharmacist involvement and regulation of medical cannabis following its availability in Arkansas	https://doi.org/10.1016/j.japh.2023.05.014	No

(continued)

(continued)

PubMed ID	First author surname	Article title	DOI number	Citation included in the study (yes/no)
37199833	Wang	Assessment of clinical outcomes in patients with fibromyalgia: analysis from the UK medical cannabis registry	https://doi.org/10.1002/brb3.3072	No
37191563	Aladeen	Medical cannabis in the treatment of Parkinson's Disease	https://doi.org/10.1097/WNF.0000000000000550	Yes—article was behind a paywall and could not be accessed
37172308	Anis	Licensed medical cannabis use in Gilles de la Tourette Syndrome: a retrospective long-term follow-up	https://doi.org/10.1089/can.2022.0281	Yes—article was behind a paywall and could not be accessed
37168830	Jankie	A cross-sectional survey of prospective healthcare professionals' knowledge, attitudes and perceptions of medical cannabis	https://doi.org/10.1016/j.rcsop.2023.100275	No
37159196	Arkell	Assessment of medical cannabis and health-related quality of life	https://doi.org/10.1001/jamanetworkopen.2023.12522	No
37155939	Pav	Public knowledge, perceptions, and behavioral intention regarding medical cannabis in Belgium	https://doi.org/10.1080/02791072.2023.2209893	No
37155681	Dekeseredy	Using medical cannabis for chronic pain: a social-ecological framework	https://doi.org/10.1089/can.2023.0016	No
37151922	Mansell	Medical cannabis in schools: the experiences of caregivers	https://doi.org/10.1093/pch/pxac099	No
37151920	Mansell	Medical cannabis in schools: a qualitative study on the experiences of clinicians	https://doi.org/10.1093/pch/pxac110	Yes
37147415	Butler	The information-seeking behavior and unmet knowledge needs of older medicinal cannabis consumers in Canada: a qualitative descriptive study	https://doi.org/10.1007/s40266-023-01030-8	No
37130724	Aprikian	Medical cannabis is effective for cancer-related pain: Quebec cannabis registry results	https://doi.org/10.1136/spcare-2022-004003	No
37130467	Myers	Assessing the diagnostic utility of the Cannabis use disorder identification test—revised (CUDIT-R) among veterans with medical and non-medical cannabis use	https://doi.org/10.1016/j.drugalcdep.2023.109876	No

(continued)

(continued)

PubMed ID	First author surname	Article title	DOI number	Citation included in the study (yes/no)
37124080	Jugl	Climbing the evidence Pyramid: dosing considerations for medical cannabis in the management of chronic pain	https://doi.org/10.1159/000530251	No
37122648	Alharbi	Knowledge, perception, and beliefs of Saudi physicians at King Abdulaziz Medical City, Riyadh related to medical cannabis: literature review and a cross-sectional survey	https://doi.org/10.4103/jfmpc.jfmpc_1856_22	Yes
37116158	Sukrueangkul	Factors associated with demand for medical cannabis use among breast cancer patients in Northern Thailand: a cross-sectional study	https://doi.org/10.31557/APJCP.2023.24.4.1351	No
37107712	Efron	Medicinal cannabis for paediatric developmental, behavioural and mental health disorders	https://doi.org/10.3390/ijerph20085430	Yes
37098170	Kruger	Physicians' attitudes and practices regarding cannabis and recommending medical cannabis use	https://doi.org/10.1089/can.2022.0324	Yes—article was behind a paywall and could not be accessed
37090897	Suraev	Medical cannabis use patterns for sleep disorders in Australia: results of the cross-sectional CAMS-20 survey	https://doi.org/10.2147/NSS.S390583	Yes
37089954	Clarke	The evolving culture of medical cannabis in Canada for the management of chronic pain	https://doi.org/10.3389/fphar.2023.1153584	No
37078172	Erridge	Letter to the editor: reflections on the future of medical cannabis research for depression	https://doi.org/10.1080/14737175.2023.2203862	No
37077169	O'Neill	Medicinal Cannabis and implications for workplace health and safety: scoping review of systematic reviews	https://doi.org/10.1177/21650799231157086	No
37068050	Modesto-Lowe	Cross-national reflections on medicinal cannabis and depression	https://doi.org/10.1080/14737175.2023.2203861	No
37057257	Schubert	Medicinal cannabis for Australian patients with chronic refractory pain including arthritis	https://doi.org/10.1177/2049463722114711 5	No
37021592	Tait	Clinical outcome data of chronic pain patients treated with cannabis-based oils and dried flower from the UK medical cannabis registry	https://doi.org/10.1080/14737175.2023.2195551	No

(continued)

(continued)

PubMed ID	First author surname	Article title	DOI number	Citation included in the study (yes/no)
37019380	Kane	Institutional policy consideration for medical cannabis	https://doi.org/10.1016/j.japh.2023.03.010	No
37007688	Kliuk-Ben Bassat	Medical cannabis for pain management in patients undergoing chronic hemodialysis: randomized, double-blind, cross-over, feasibility study	https://doi.org/10.1093/ckj/sfac275	No
36978185	Zolotov	"It doesn't make any sense to even try": the disruptive impact of COVID-19's first wave on people with chronic pain using medical cannabis in New York	https://doi.org/10.1186/s42238-023-00180-1	No
36974286	Fones	Erratum to "hand surgery patient perspectives on medical cannabis: a survey of over 600 patients" [Journal of Hand Surgery Global Online 5 (2023) 102–107]	https://doi.org/10.1016/j.jhsg.2023.02.001	No
34283433	Bodine MKemp	Medical cannabis use in oncology		No
36965450	Russo	Enantioseparation of chiral phytocannabinoids in medicinal cannabis	https://doi.org/10.1016/j.chromb.2023.123682	No
36961410	Zhang	Factors associated with medical cannabis use after certification: a three-month longitudinal study	https://doi.org/10.1089/can.2022.0248	No
36960460	Cooke	Development of cannabis use disorder in medical cannabis users: a 9-month follow-up of a randomized clinical trial testing effects of medical cannabis card ownership	https://doi.org/10.3389/fpsyt.2023.1083334	No
36952564	Shim	Lessons from 20 years of medical cannabis use in Canada	https://doi.org/10.1371/journal.pone.0271079	No
36949852	Li	Use of non-medical cannabis in epilepsy: a scoping review	https://doi.org/10.3389/fneur.2023.1132106	No
36941425	White	Perceived safety and effectiveness of cannabis and other types of pain treatments among adults with chronic noncancer pain in U.S. States with medical cannabis programs	https://doi.org/10.1007/s11606-023-08163-x	No

(continued)

(continued)

PubMed ID	First author surname	Article title	DOI number	Citation included in the study (yes/no)
36937098	Reiman	Medical cannabis identity and public health paternalism	https://doi.org/10.1016/j.puhip.2023.100372	No
36933893	Myran	Access to legal cannabis market in Canada over the four years following non-medical cannabis legalisation	https://doi.org/10.1111/dar.13650	No
36924465	Lake	Shifts in medical cannabis use in Canada during the COVID-19 pandemic	https://doi.org/10.24095/hpcdp.43.3.02	No
36914573	Lewis	Media framing of causes, risks, and policy solutions for cannabis-impaired driving: does medical versus non-medical cannabis context matter?	https://doi.org/10.1080/10410236.2023.2187956	No
36903921	Peterswald	Moving away from 12:12; the effect of different photoperiods on biomass yield and Cannabinoids in medicinal cannabis	https://doi.org/10.3390/plants12051061	No
36897501	Hameed	Medical cannabis for chronic nonmalignant pain management	https://doi.org/10.1007/s11916-023-01101-w	No
36896798	Cohn	Seeing is believing: how cannabis marketing exposure is associated with cannabis use attitudes and behavior in a permissive medical cannabis policy environment	https://doi.org/10.1111/ajad.13390	No
36893511	N S Gendy	Prevalence of cannabis use disorder among individuals using medical cannabis at admission to inpatient treatment for substance use disorders	https://doi.org/10.1016/j.addbeh.2023.107667	No
36888538	Gething	Stakeholders' decisions and preferences for the provision and use of medicinal cannabis: a scoping review	https://doi.org/10.1089/can.2022.0115	No
36854217	Meier	The effects of the 4/20 cannabis holiday and adult-use cannabis legalization on medical cannabis sales and medical cannabis patient registration in Arizona	https://doi.org/10.1016/j.drugpo.2023.103974	No
36848456	Olsson	An observational study of safety and clinical outcome measures across patient groups in the United Kingdom medical cannabis registry	https://doi.org/10.1080/17512433.2023.2183841	No

(continued)

(continued)

PubMed ID	First author surname	Article title	DOI number	Citation included in the study (yes/no)
36836018	Morris	A retrospective medical record review of adults with non-cancer diagnoses prescribed medicinal cannabis	https://doi.org/10.3390/jcm12041483	No
36814687	Treyer	Phytochemical comparison of medicinal cannabis extracts and study of their CYP-mediated interactions with Coumarinic oral anticoagulants	https://doi.org/10.1159/000528465	No
36809569	Lim	What is the hype on #MedicinalCannabis in the United States? A content analysis of medicinal cannabis tweets	https://doi.org/10.1111/dar.13618	No
36807590	Gliksberg	Negative experiences of patients using medicinal cannabis: a systematic review of qualitative studies	https://doi.org/10.1111/jocn.16653	Yes
36803620	Bapir	Comparing the effects of medical cannabis for chronic pain patients with and without co-morbid anxiety: a cohort study	https://doi.org/10.1080/14737175.2023.2181696	Yes
36800328	Wolfe	Impacts of medical and non-medical cannabis on the health of older adults: findings from a scoping review of the literature	https://doi.org/10.1371/journal.pone.0281826	No
36798752	Ahrens	Prevalence and association of non-medical cannabis use with post-procedural healthcare utilisation in patients undergoing surgery or interventional procedures: a retrospective cohort study	https://doi.org/10.1016/j.eclinm.2023.101831	No
36795103	Hallinan	Corrigendum to: use of electronic medical records to monitor the safe and effective prescribing of medicinal cannabis: is it feasible?	https://doi.org/10.1071/PY22054_CO	No
36793224	Canals	Patient reported outcomes using medical cannabis for managing pain in charcot-marie-tooth disease	https://doi.org/10.1177/10499091231158388	No
36787207	Auguste	Self-reported impacts of recreational and medicinal cannabis use on driving ability and amount of wait time before driving	https://doi.org/10.1080/15389588.2023.2172679	No

(continued)

(continued)

PubMed ID	First author surname	Article title	DOI number	Citation included in the study (yes/no)
36762986	Tait	UK medical cannabis registry: a patient evaluation	https://doi.org/10.1080/15360288.2023.2174633	No
36741572	Nacasch	Medical cannabis for treatment-resistant combat PTSD	https://doi.org/10.3389/fpsyt.2022.1014630	Yes
36722292	Nicholas	UK medical cannabis registry: assessment of clinical outcomes in patients with headache disorders	https://doi.org/10.1080/14737175.2023.2174017	No
36720084	Nguyen	Changes in medical cannabis use after recreational cannabis legalization in Canada	https://doi.org/10.1089/can.2022.0227	No
36716026	Nguyen	Changes in prescribed opioid dosages among patients receiving medical cannabis for chronic pain, New York State, 2017–2019	https://doi.org/10.1001/jamanetworkopen.2022.54573	No
36704391	Fones	Hand surgery patient perspectives on medical cannabis: a survey of over 600 patients	https://doi.org/10.1016/j.jhsg.2022.02.009	No
36672666	Hajjar	A longitudinal observational study of medical cannabis use and polypharmacy among patients presenting to dispensaries in Pennsylvania	https://doi.org/10.3390/biomedicines11010158	No
36650442	Rosenbaek	GPs' prescription patterns, experience, and attitudes towards medicinal cannabis-a nationwide survey at the early stage of the Danish test scheme	https://doi.org/10.1186/s12875-023-01971-4	Yes
36641008	Jafri	Medical cannabis for insomnia in a patient with advanced breast cancer	https://doi.org/10.1016/j.jpainsymman.2023.01.002	No
36638694	Yana	Risk of depressive disorders associated with medical cannabis authorization: a propensity score matched cohort study	https://doi.org/10.1016/j.psychres.2022.115047	No
36623871	Eymery	Linking medicinal cannabis to autotaxin-lysophosphatidic acid signaling	https://doi.org/10.26508/lsa.202201595	No
36615107	Christensen	Clinical research evidence supporting administration and dosing recommendations of medicinal cannabis as analgesic in cancer patients	https://doi.org/10.3390/jcm12010307	No

(continued)

(continued)

PubMed ID	First author surname	Article title	DOI number	Citation included in the study (yes/no)
36609049	Yang	Medical cannabis in hand surgery: a review of the current evidence	https://doi.org/10.1016/j.jhsa.2022.11.008	No
36607641	Bicket	Use of cannabis and other pain treatments among adults with chronic pain in US States with medical cannabis programs	https://doi.org/10.1001/jamanetworkopen.2022.49797	No
36605951	Garrido	Exogenous application of stress-related signaling molecules affect growth and cannabinoid accumulation in medical cannabis (*Cannabis sativa* L.)	https://doi.org/10.3389/fpls.2022.1082554	No
36589471	Boury	Developments and changes in primary public health outcome indicators associated with the legalization of non-medical cannabis use and supply in Canada (2018): a comprehensive overview	https://doi.org/10.1007/s11469-022-00986-9	No
36579921	Vigano	The Quebec cannabis registry: investigating the safety and effectiveness of medical cannabis	https://doi.org/10.1089/can.2022.0041	No
36573268	Mangoo	Assessment of clinical outcomes of medicinal cannabis therapy for depression: analysis from the UK medical cannabis registry	https://doi.org/10.1080/14737175.2022.2161894	Yes
36562418	Dalavaye	The effect of medical cannabis in inflammatory bowel disease: analysis from the UK medical cannabis registry	https://doi.org/10.1080/17474124.2022.2161046	No
36555842	Seifalian	Dysmenorrhoea: can medicinal cannabis bring new hope for a collective group of women suffering in pain, globally?	https://doi.org/10.3390/ijms232416201	No
36540576	Ng	Surveying Canadian pain physicians' attitudes and beliefs regarding medical Cannabis for chronic noncancer pain: a qualitative study	https://doi.org/10.2147/JPR.S382589	Yes
36539991	Ried	Medicinal cannabis improves sleep in adults with insomnia: a randomised double-blind placebo-controlled crossover study	https://doi.org/10.1111/jsr.13793	Yes

(continued)

(continued)

PubMed ID	First author surname	Article title	DOI number	Citation included in the study (yes/no)
36539215	Erridge	Clinical outcome data of children treated with cannabis-based medicinal products for treatment resistant epilepsy-analysis from the UK medical cannabis registry	https://doi.org/10.1055/a-2002-2119	Yes
36535195	Waissengrin	The use of medical cannabis concomitantly with immune checkpoint inhibitors in non-small cell lung cancer: a sigh of relief?	https://doi.org/10.1016/j.ejca.2022.11.022	No
36529730	Bawa	Knowledge, experiences, and attitudes of Australian general practitioners towards medicinal cannabis: a 2021–2022 survey	https://doi.org/10.1186/s12875-022-01946-x	Yes
36514999	Willow	Towards dsRNA-integrated protection of medical cannabis crops: considering human safety, recent- and developing RNAi methods, and research inroads	https://doi.org/10.1002/ps.7323	No
36506781	Hard	Medical cannabis laws and adolescent alcohol use initiation	https://doi.org/10.26828/cannabis/2022.03.001	No
36503404	Pillai	Assessment of clinical outcomes in patients with post-traumatic stress disorder: analysis from the UK medical cannabis registry	https://doi.org/10.1080/14737175.2022.2155139	Yes
34662076	Bains SMukhdomi	Medicinal cannabis for treatment of chronic pain		No
36484577	DiGuiseppi	Egocentric network characteristics and cannabis use in a sample of young adult medical cannabis patients and nonpatient users	https://doi.org/10.15288/jsad.21-00286	No
36459627	Malík	Selective cytotoxicity of medical cannabis (*Cannabis sativa* L.) extracts across the whole vegetation cycle under various hydroponic and nutritional treatments	https://doi.org/10.1089/can.2022.0243	No
36448002	Kalaba	Longitudinal relationship between the introduction of medicinal cannabis and polypharmacy: an Australian real-world evidence study	https://doi.org/10.1155/2022/8535207	No
36446995	Bawa	A cross-sectional survey exploring the knowledge, experiences and attitudes of Australian pharmacists toward medicinal cannabis	https://doi.org/10.1007/s11096-022-01519-z	Yes

(continued)

(continued)

PubMed ID	First author surname	Article title	DOI number	Citation included in the study (yes/no)
36445409	Schubert	Medicinal cannabis for patients with chronic non-cancer pain: analysis of safety and concomitant medications	https://doi.org/10.1093/ijpp/riac073	No
36443110	Armstrong	Relationships between sales of legal medical cannabis and alcohol in Canada	https://doi.org/10.1016/j.healthpol.2022.11.012	No
36435953	Nayak	Medical cannabis-related stigma: cancer survivors' perspectives	https://doi.org/10.1007/s11764-022-01297-7	No
36429798	Duan	State T21, restrictions on flavored E-cigarette products, and non-medical cannabis sales legalization in relation to young adult reports of vape shop age verification and product offerings: a multilevel analysis	https://doi.org/10.3390/ijerph192215079	No
36413342	Aron	Effects of medical cannabis certification on hospital use by individuals with sickle cell disease	https://doi.org/10.1089/can.2022.0136	Yes—article was behind a paywall and could not be accessed
36405915	Schlag	The value of real world evidence: the case of medical cannabis	https://doi.org/10.3389/fpsyt.2022.1027159	No
36399996	Erridge	Patient priorities for research: a focus group study of UK medical cannabis patients	https://doi.org/10.1016/j.ctcp.2022.101693	Yes
36399463	Vickery	A large Australian longitudinal cohort registry demonstrates sustained safety and efficacy of oral medicinal cannabis for at least two years	https://doi.org/10.1371/journal.pone.0272241	No
36383424	Montmeat	Sex differences in medical cannabis-related adverse effects? Do not forget the context!	https://doi.org/10.1097/j.pain.0000000000002771	No
36380639	Rozmann	Public perception of guilt and deserved punishment in medical cannabis diversion	https://doi.org/10.1111/dar.13579	No
36379690	Gurgenci	Medicinal cannabis in palliative medicine: lessons learnt from randomised controlled trials	https://doi.org/10.1136/spcare-2022-004035	No
36377286	Jochen	School nurse perspectives of medical cannabis policy in K-12 schools: an exploratory descriptive study	https://doi.org/10.1177/10598405221136288	No

(continued)

(continued)

PubMed ID	First author surname	Article title	DOI number	Citation included in the study (yes/no)
36367871	Erku	From growers to patients: multi-stakeholder views on the use of, and access to medicinal cannabis in Australia	https://doi.org/10.1371/journal.pone.0277355	No
36367574	Dahlgren	Increased white matter coherence following three and six months of medical cannabis treatment	https://doi.org/10.1089/can.2022.0097	No
36346322	Kulpa	Serum markers of bone turnover following controlled administration of two medical cannabis products in healthy adults	https://doi.org/10.1089/can.2022.0181	No
36342913	Barchel	Use of medical cannabis in patients with gilles de la tourette's syndrome in a real-world setting	https://doi.org/10.1089/can.2022.0112	Yes—article was behind a paywall and could not be accessed
36342776	Ajrawat	Medical cannabis use and inflammatory cytokines and chemokines among adult chronic pain patients	https://doi.org/10.1089/can.2022.0143	No
36335552	Olson	'What price do you put on your health?': Medical cannabis, financial toxicity and patient perspectives on medication access in advanced cancer	https://doi.org/10.1111/hex.13642	No
36317603	Van Boxem	Conflicting recommendations: a labyrinth for the clinician and patients: a comment to Eisenberg's et al. "medical cannabis for chronic pain"	https://doi.org/10.1002/ejp.2050	No
36309761	Erridge	Medical cannabis, CBD wellness products and public awareness of evolving regulations in the United Kingdom	https://doi.org/10.1186/s42238-022-00165-6	No
36271334	Mekrungrongwong	Self-perceived knowledge, attitudes, and training needs regarding medical cannabis among health care providers and health volunteers in district health systems, Phitsanulok Province	https://doi.org/10.1186/s12875-022-01877-7	No
36251467	Awal	Medical Cannabis in Canadian schools: a scoping review of existing policies	https://doi.org/10.1089/can.2021.0199	No
36249785	Stolar	Medical cannabis for the treatment of comorbid symptoms in children with autism spectrum disorder: an interim analysis of biochemical safety	https://doi.org/10.3389/fphar.2022.977484	No

(continued)

(continued)

PubMed ID	First author surname	Article title	DOI number	Citation included in the study (yes/no)
36247643	Danziger	Too dense or not too dense: higher planting density reduces cannabinoid uniformity but increases yield/area in drug-type medical cannabis	https://doi.org/10.3389/fpls.2022.713481	No
36227025	Greywoode	Medical cannabis use patterns and adverse effects in inflammatory bowel disease	https://doi.org/10.1097/MCG.0000000000001782	Yes—article was behind a paywall and could not be accessed
36204633	Skala	Medical cannabis dimethyl ether, ethanol and butane extracts inhibit the in vitro growth of bacteria and dermatophytes causing common skin diseases	https://doi.org/10.3389/fmicb.2022.953092	No
36200224	Ramos Atance	Can we increase risk perception among medical cannabis users?	https://doi.org/10.20882/adicciones.1656	No
36196529	Barré	Exploring the medical cannabis prescribing behaviours of French general practitioners	https://doi.org/10.1111/dar.13547	No
36192811	Wieghorst	The effect of medical cannabis on cognitive functions: a systematic review	https://doi.org/10.1186/s13643-022-02073-5	No
36182689	Sznitman	Posttraumatic stress disorder, sleep and medical cannabis treatment: a daily diary study	https://doi.org/10.1016/j.janxdis.2022.102632	Yes
36172004	Ross	Increasing access to safe medical cannabis: establishment of a medical cannabis program in a safety-net academic medical center	https://doi.org/10.1056/cat.21.0373	No
36171626	Bania	Shifts in therapeutic practices and decline of medicinal cannabis in Indian North-Eastern Frontier (1826–1925)	https://doi.org/10.1186/s42238-022-00159-4	No
36168378	Clobes	Differences in attitudes toward medical cannabis with humanized patient scenarios	https://doi.org/10.7759/cureus.28354	No
36168342	Jacobs	Medical students' attitudes, knowledge, and beliefs about medical cannabis: a qualitative descriptive study	https://doi.org/10.7759/cureus.28336	No
36168127	Pritchett	Medical cannabis patients report improvements in health functioning and reductions in opiate use	https://doi.org/10.1080/10826084.2022.2107673	No

(continued)

(continued)

PubMed ID	First author surname	Article title	DOI number	Citation included in the study (yes/no)
36165867	Birenboim	Use of near-infrared spectroscopy for the classification of medicinal cannabis cultivars and the prediction of their cannabinoid and terpene contents	https://doi.org/10.1016/j.phytochem.2022.113445	No
36165188	Myran	Changes in health harms due to cannabis following legalisation of non-medical cannabis in Canada in context of cannabis commercialisation: a scoping review	https://doi.org/10.1111/dar.13546	No
36159065	Erridge	Clinical outcome analysis of patients with autism spectrum disorder: analysis from the UK medical cannabis registry	https://doi.org/10.1177/20451253221116240	Yes
36147312	Garcia-Romeu	Online survey of medicinal cannabis users: qualitative analysis of patient-level data	https://doi.org/10.3389/fphar.2022.965535	Yes
36131299	MacNair	Medical cannabis authorization patterns, safety, and associated effects in older adults	https://doi.org/10.1186/s42238-022-00158-5	No
36122285	Gómez-García	Medical cannabis: critical points for clinical application	https://doi.org/10.7705/biomedica.6468	No
36121021	Trojan	Assessment of delta-9-tetrahydrocannabinol (THC) in saliva and blood after oral administration of medical cannabis with respect to its effect on driving abilities	https://doi.org/10.33549/physiolres.934907	No
36098574	Townsend	Perspectives of orthopedic patients on medical cannabis: a survey of more than 2500 patients	https://doi.org/10.3928/01477447-20220907-05	No
36091749	Brusa	Editorial: medicinal cannabis: evolution of therapeutic use, future approaches and other implications	https://doi.org/10.3389/fphar.2022.999068	No
36064621	Olson	Using a qualitative sub-study to inform the design and delivery of randomised controlled trials on medicinal cannabis for symptom relief in patients with advanced cancer	https://doi.org/10.1186/s13063-022-06691-1	No
36055965	Cheng	Healthcare professionals' perspectives on the use of medicinal cannabis to manage chronic pain: a systematic search and narrative review	https://doi.org/10.1111/papr.13161	Yes

(continued)

(continued)

PubMed ID	First author surname	Article title	DOI number	Citation included in the study (yes/no)
36055728	Burnett	Policy ahead of the science: medical cannabis laws versus scientific evidence	https://doi.org/10.1016/j.psc.2022.05.002	No
36017106	Nussbaum	Practices and perspectives on medical cannabis and cannabinoids: a survey of the national psoriasis foundation medical advisory board	https://doi.org/10.1016/j.jdin.2022.07.001	No
36011488	Hallinan	The rise and rise of medicinal cannabis, what now? Medicinal cannabis prescribing in Australia 2017–2022	https://doi.org/10.3390/ijerph19169853	No
35994572	Idan	Evaluation of immune response to anti-COVID-19 booster in cancer patients and chronic medical cannabis users and its association with circulating Eosinophils levels	https://doi.org/10.1002/cac2.12353	No
35991815	Bandawe	Medical cannabis and cannabidiol: a new harvest for Malawi	https://doi.org/10.4314/mmj.v34i2.10	No
35977118	Hughes	Medical cannabis or cannabinoids for chronic pain: BMJ rapid recommendation		No
35950052	Abelev	Medicinal cannabis for the treatment of chronic refractory pain: an investigation of the adverse event profile and health-related quality of life impact of an oral formulation	https://doi.org/10.1159/000521492	No
35944268	Uziel	Solid-state microwave drying for medical cannabis inflorescences: a rapid and controlled alternative to traditional drying	https://doi.org/10.1089/can.2022.0051	No
35927928	Hallinan	Use of electronic medical records to monitor the safe and effective prescribing of medicinal cannabis: is it feasible?	https://doi.org/10.1071/PY22054	No
35926992	Zeraatkar	Long-term and serious harms of medical cannabis and cannabinoids for chronic pain: a systematic review of non-randomised studies	https://doi.org/10.1136/bmjopen-2021-054282	No
35917529	Dahlgren	A survey of medical cannabis use during perimenopause and postmenopause	https://doi.org/10.1097/GME.0000000000002018	No

(continued)

(continued)

PubMed ID	First author surname	Article title	DOI number	Citation included in the study (yes/no)
35908759	Berger	Medicinal cannabis for the treatment of anxiety disorders	https://doi.org/10.31128/AJGP-04-21-5936	No
35907959	Lintzeris	Medical cannabis use in Australia: consumer experiences from the online cannabis as medicine survey 2020 (CAMS-20)	https://doi.org/10.1186/s12954-022-00666-w	No
35876631	Sotoodeh	Predictors of pain reduction among fibromyalgia patients using medical cannabis: a long-term prospective cohort study	https://doi.org/10.1002/acr.24985	No
35866679	Zongo	Incidence and predictors of cannabis-related poisoning and mental and behavioral disorders among patients with medical cannabis authorization: a cohort study	https://doi.org/10.1080/10826084.2022.2102193	No
35851324	Carnide	Cannabis use and workplace cannabis availability, perceptions and policies among Canadian workers: a comparison before and after the legalisation of non-medical cannabis	https://doi.org/10.1136/oemed-2022-108316	No
35838430	Wardell	Correlates of self-reported medicinal cannabis use for physical health, mental health, and sleep-related conditions in a population-based survey of Canadian youth		No
35821596	Trangenstein	Commentary on Gunadi et al.: opportunities to design more policy-relevant evaluations of non-medical cannabis legalization	https://doi.org/10.1111/add.15984	No
35820952	Macedo	Online information on medical cannabis is not always aligned with scientific evidence and may raise unrealistic expectations	https://doi.org/10.1186/s42238-022-00145-w	No
35812569	Jacobs	Exploratory factor analysis of medical students' perceptions of medical cannabis scale	https://doi.org/10.7759/cureus.25749	No
35796526	Mangual-Pérez	Patient experience and perspective on medical cannabis as an alternative for musculoskeletal pain management	https://doi.org/10.5435/JAAOSGlobal-D-22-00055	No

(continued)

(continued)

PubMed ID	First author surname	Article title	DOI number	Citation included in the study (yes/no)
35773908	Wongkongdech	Symptom management and quality of life of palliative cancer patients after being administered with thai medicinal cannabis	https://doi.org/10.3233/SHTI220762	No
35760442	Wise	Medical cannabis: allow GPs to prescribe as part of national trial, review urges	https://doi.org/10.1136/bmj.o1567	No
35749740	Nathan	Assessing efficacy and use patterns of medical cannabis for symptom management in elderly cancer patients	https://doi.org/10.1177/10499091221110217	No
35733629	Poli	Promising health benefits of adjuvant Acmella and Zingiber extracts combined with coenzyme Q10 phytosomes, supplementation in chronic pain treated with medical cannabis: a prospective and open-label clinical study	https://doi.org/10.1155/2022/7099161	No
35728125	Withanarachchie	Assessing progress with the implementation of the New Zealand medicinal cannabis scheme		No
35723729	Kasvis	Sex differences exist in the perceived relief of cancer symptoms with medical cannabis: results from the Quebec cannabis registry	https://doi.org/10.1007/s00520-022-07193-1	No
35720524	Saloner	Nitrogen source matters: high NH(4)/NO(3) ratio reduces cannabinoids, terpenoids, and yield in medical cannabis	https://doi.org/10.3389/fpls.2022.830224	No
35712276	Fortin	Medical cannabis: toward a new policy and health model for an ancient medicine	https://doi.org/10.3389/fpubh.2022.904291	No
35711271	Okusanya	Medical cannabis for the treatment of migraine in adults: a review of the evidence	https://doi.org/10.3389/fneur.2022.871187	No
35710586	de Souza	Medical cannabis regulation: an overview of models around the world with emphasis on the Brazilian scenario	https://doi.org/10.1186/s42238-022-00142-z	No
35701148	Gurgenci	Research agenda for medical cannabis in palliative care	https://doi.org/10.1136/bmjspcare-2022-003747	No
35698183	Holman	Healthcare provider and medical cannabis patient communication regarding referral and medication substitution: the Canadian context	https://doi.org/10.1186/s42238-022-00141-0	No

(continued)

(continued)

PubMed ID	First author surname	Article title	DOI number	Citation included in the study (yes/no)
35696691	Boehnke	U.S. Trends in registration for medical cannabis and reasons for use from 2016 to 2020: an observational study	https://doi.org/10.7326/M22-0217	No
35691014	Ellis	Medical cannabis and automobile accidents: Evidence from auto insurance	https://doi.org/10.1002/hec.4553	No
35679600	Tung	Cancer patients' experiences with and perspectives on the medicinal cannabis "high"	https://doi.org/10.1089/jpm.2022.0119	No
35669038	Aviram	The effectiveness and safety of medical cannabis for treating cancer related symptoms in oncology patients	https://doi.org/10.3389/fpain.2022.861037	No
35640046	Clary	Weeding out the stigma: older veterans in Illinois share their experiences using medical cannabis	https://doi.org/10.1080/02791072.2022.2082901	No
35636009	Lo Faro	Ultra-high-performance liquid chromatography-tandem mass spectrometry assay for quantifying THC, CBD and their metabolites in hair. Application to patients treated with medical cannabis	https://doi.org/10.1016/j.jpba.2022.114841	No
35622192	Trangenstein	Typology of adolescents exposed to non-medical cannabis marketing and associations with consumption patterns	https://doi.org/10.1007/s11121-022-01378-0	No
35620292	MacPhail	Medicinal cannabis prescribing in Australia: an analysis of trends over the first five years	https://doi.org/10.3389/fphar.2022.885655	No
35620248	Aviram	Long-term effectiveness and safety of medical cannabis administered through the metered-dose Syqe Inhaler	https://doi.org/10.1097/PR9.0000000000001011	No
35620050	Mauro	Daily cannabis use, cannabis use disorder, and any medical cannabis use among US adults: Associations within racial, ethnic, and sexual minoritized identities in a changing policy context	https://doi.org/10.1016/j.pmedr.2022.101822	No
35619867	Jacobs	Predictors of medical students' perceptions about medical cannabis	https://doi.org/10.7759/cureus.24390	No
35616591	Rampakakis	Medical cannabis use by rheumatology patients in routine clinical care: results from The Ontario best practices research initiative	https://doi.org/10.55563/clinexprheumatol/b85xu5	Yes—article was behind a paywall and could not be accessed

(continued)

(continued)

PubMed ID	First author surname	Article title	DOI number	Citation included in the study (yes/no)
35614947	Anil	Medical cannabis activity against inflammation: active compounds and modes of action	https://doi.org/10.3389/fphar.2022.908198	No
35611178	Maddison	Is there a place for medicinal cannabis in treating patients with sleep disorders? What we know so far	https://doi.org/10.2147/NSS.S340949	No
35604868	Manoharan	Exploring the medical cannabis prescribing behaviours of New Zealand physicians	https://doi.org/10.1111/dar.13476	Yes
35604691	Lapham	Comparison of medical cannabis use reported on a confidential survey versus documented in the electronic health record among primary care patients	https://doi.org/10.1001/jamanetworkopen.2022.11677	No
35598566	Sachedina	Medical cannabis use in Canada and its impact on anxiety and depression: A retrospective study	https://doi.org/10.1016/j.psychres.2022.114573	Yes
35585574	Sokratous	Attitudes, beliefs and knowledge about medical cannabis among nurses and midwives in Cyprus: a cross-sectional descriptive correlational study	https://doi.org/10.1186/s12912-022-00887-1	No
35576357	Shoshan	Medical Cannabis for gynecologic pain conditions: a systematic review	https://doi.org/10.1097/AOG.0000000000004777	No
35571129	Lacroix	What do we know about medical cannabis in neurological disorders and what are the next steps?	https://doi.org/10.3389/fphar.2022.883987	No
35532992	Minhas	Letter to the editor: the need for equitable health care among medical cannabis patients in Canada	https://doi.org/10.1089/can.2022.0084	No
35529444	Ortiz	Medicinal cannabis and central nervous system disorders	https://doi.org/10.3389/fphar.2022.881810	No
35519806	Naim-Feil	Empirical evaluation of inflorescences' morphological attributes for yield optimization of medicinal cannabis cultivars	https://doi.org/10.3389/fpls.2022.858519	No
35512367	Kurtzman	Are patients who trust their providers more likely to use medical cannabis?	https://doi.org/10.1177/10499091221097090	No
35488381	Hulaihel	Medical cannabis and stigma: a qualitative study with patients living with chronic pain	https://doi.org/10.1111/jocn.16340	No

(continued)

(continued)

PubMed ID	First author surname	Article title	DOI number	Citation included in the study (yes/no)
35485690	Sukrueangkul	Attitudes and beliefs of cancer patients demanding medical cannabis use in North Thailand	https://doi.org/10.31557/APJCP.2022.23.4.1309	No
35442765	Eyal	Vapor pressure, vaping, and corrections to misconceptions related to medical cannabis' active pharmaceutical ingredients' physical properties and compositions	https://doi.org/10.1089/can.2021.0173	No
35432432	Malík	Amino acid supplementation as a biostimulant in medical cannabis (*Cannabis sativa* L.) plant nutrition	https://doi.org/10.3389/fpls.2022.868350	No
35432009	Rubin-Kahana	Medical cannabis and past-year cannabis use disorder among adult recreational users in the United States: results from a nationally representative sample	https://doi.org/10.3389/fpsyt.2022.836908	No
35412332	Jerushalmi	Members of the fusarium oxysporum complex causing wilt symptoms in medical cannabis in Israel, Italy, and North America comprise a polyphyletic assemblage	https://doi.org/10.1094/PDIS-01-22-0155-RE	No
35394802	Patell	Oncology fellows' clinical discussions, perceived knowledge, and formal training regarding medical cannabis use: a national survey study	https://doi.org/10.1200/OP.21.00714	No
35392181	Kendzor	Characteristics of adults with a medical cannabis license, reasons for use, and perceptions of benefit following medical cannabis legalization in Oklahoma	https://doi.org/10.1016/j.pmedr.2022.101777	No
35387635	Cunningham	Availability of medical cannabis services by racial, social, and geographic characteristics of neighborhoods in New York: a cross-sectional study	https://doi.org/10.1186/s12889-022-13076-1	No
35382939	Santarossa	Medical cannabis use in Canadians with multiple sclerosis	https://doi.org/10.1016/j.msard.2022.103638	Yes—article was behind a paywall and could not be accessed
35363933	Eisenberg	Medicinal cannabis for chronic pain: the bermuda triangle of low-quality studies, countless meta-analyses and conflicting recommendations	https://doi.org/10.1002/ejp.1946	No

(continued)

(continued)

PubMed ID	First author surname	Article title	DOI number	Citation included in the study (yes/no)
35360989	Razmovski-Naumovski	Efficacy of medicinal cannabis for appetite-related symptoms in people with cancer: a systematic review	https://doi.org/10.1177/02692163221083437	No
35343818	Siani-Rose	The potential of salivary lipid-based cannabis-responsive biomarkers to evaluate medical cannabis treatment in children with autism spectrum disorder	https://doi.org/10.1089/can.2021.0224	No
35338476	Veit	Quality requirements for medicinal cannabis and respective products in the European Union—status quo	https://doi.org/10.1055/a-1808-9708	No
35337156	Malach	Medical cannabis in pediatric oncology: friend or foe?	https://doi.org/10.3390/ph15030359	No
35331185	Vinette	Routes of administration, reasons for use, and approved indications of medical cannabis in oncology: a scoping review	https://doi.org/10.1186/s12885-022-09378-7	No
35319304	Lazris	Integrated medical cannabis consultations in a palliative care program: policies, procedures, and progress after six years of practice	https://doi.org/10.1089/jpm.2021.0577	No
35310886	Anis	Medical cannabis for Gilles de la Tourette syndrome: an open-label prospective study	https://doi.org/10.1155/2022/5141773	Yes
35308110	Abalo	Between facts and ambiguity: discourses on medical cannabis in Swedish newspapers	https://doi.org/10.1177/1455072521996997	No
35292477	Gunning	Clinician views on and ethics priorities for authorizing medical cannabis in the care of children and youth in Canada: a qualitative study	https://doi.org/10.9778/cmajo.20210239	Yes
35289010	Lorenzetti	The iCannToolkit: a tool to embrace measurement of medicinal and non-medicinal cannabis use across licit, illicit and cross-cultural settings	https://doi.org/10.1111/add.15855	No
35283868	Murovec	Analysis of morphological traits, cannabinoid profiles, THCAS gene sequences, and photosynthesis in wide and narrow leaflet high-Cannabidiol breeding populations of medical cannabis	https://doi.org/10.3389/fpls.2022.786161	No

(continued)

(continued)

PubMed ID	First author surname	Article title	DOI number	Citation included in the study (yes/no)
35273067		Correction: so near yet so far: why won't the UK prescribe medical cannabis?	https://doi.org/10.1136/bmjopen-2020-038687corr1	No
35268820	Al Ubeed	Post-harvest operations to generate high-quality medicinal cannabis products: a systemic review	https://doi.org/10.3390/molecules27051719	No
33760522	Dalal RKudur	Evaluation and treatment of pain with medicinal cannabis		No
35254218	Carrell	Clinical documentation of patient-reported medical cannabis use in primary care: toward scalable extraction using natural language processing methods	https://doi.org/10.1080/08897077.2021.1986767	No
35228923	Renslo	Medical cannabis use reduces opioid prescriptions in patients with osteoarthritis	https://doi.org/10.7759/cureus.21564	No
35228256	Bradley	Local regulatory systems hinder prescription of medical cannabis	https://doi.org/10.1136/bmj.o440	No
35228209	Hoeh	Doctors' support of medical cannabis: an evidential rather than moral imperative	https://doi.org/10.1136/bmj.o447	No
35225341	Sabmeethavorn	Pharmacists' perceptions and experiences of medicinal cannabis dispensing: a narrative review with a systematic approach	https://doi.org/10.1093/ijpp/riac005	Yes
35223923	Bar-Lev Schleider	Adherence, safety, and effectiveness of medical cannabis and epidemiological characteristics of the patient population: a prospective study	https://doi.org/10.3389/fmed.2022.827849	No
35223236	Greis	Medical cannabis use reduces opioid prescriptions in patients with chronic back pain	https://doi.org/10.7759/cureus.21452	No
35214123	Khoury	"The two sides of the same coin"-medical cannabis, cannabinoids and immunity: pros and cons explained	https://doi.org/10.3390/pharmaceutics14020389	No
35214031	Maggini	An optimized terpene profile for a new medical cannabis oil	https://doi.org/10.3390/pharmaceutics14020298	No
35197243		Why doctors have a moral imperative to prescribe and support medical cannabis-an essay by David Nutt	https://doi.org/10.1136/bmj.o483	No

(continued)

(continued)

PubMed ID	First author surname	Article title	DOI number	Citation included in the study (yes/no)
35193442	Brammer	Coping motives mediate the association of trauma history with problematic cannabis use in young adult medical cannabis patients and non-patient cannabis users	https://doi.org/10.1080/10826084.2022.2026970	No
35163863	Al Ubeed	A comprehensive review on the techniques for extraction of bioactive compounds from medicinal cannabis	https://doi.org/10.3390/molecules27030604	No
35162564	Sinclair	"Should I Inhale?"-Perceptions, barriers, and drivers for medicinal cannabis use amongst Australian women with primary dysmenorrhoea: a qualitative study	https://doi.org/10.3390/ijerph19031536	No
35141242	Ilan	Digital medical cannabis as market differentiator: second-generation artificial intelligence systems to improve response	https://doi.org/10.3389/fmed.2021.788777	No
35130464	Assaf	Changes in medical and non-medical cannabis use among United States adults before and during the COVID-19 pandemic	https://doi.org/10.1080/00952990.2021.2007257	No
35104069	Liang	Medical Cannabis for gynecologic pain conditions: a systematic review	https://doi.org/10.1097/AOG.0000000000004656	No
35092401	Sukrueangkul	Factors influencing demand for medical cannabis use among cancer patients in the North of Thailand	https://doi.org/10.31557/APJCP.2022.23.1.319	No
35084279	Kebede	Medicinal cannabis pharmacokinetics and potential methods of delivery	https://doi.org/10.1080/10837450.2022.2035748	No
35083541	Davis	In response to the study "a randomized trial of medical cannabis in patients with stage for cancers to assess feasibility, dose requirements, impact on pain and opioid use, safety, and overall patient's satisfaction" by Dr. Zylla and colleagues	https://doi.org/10.1007/s00520-021-06768-8	No
35073161	Lake	Selective changes in medical Cannabis use early in the COVID-19 pandemic: findings from a web-based sample of adults in the United States	https://doi.org/10.1089/can.2021.0115	No

(continued)

(continued)

PubMed ID	First author surname	Article title	DOI number	Citation included in the study (yes/no)
35073160	Ergisi	An updated analysis of clinical outcome measures across patients from the UK medical cannabis registry	https://doi.org/10.1089/can.2021.0145	No
35067772	Zloto	Medical cannabis oil for benign essential blepharospasm: a prospective, randomized controlled pilot study	https://doi.org/10.1007/s00417-021-05533-1	No
35138770	Slawek DWhitley	Therapeutic use of medical cannabis in New York State		No
35051158	Benedict	Medical cannabis used as an alternative treatment for chronic pain demonstrates reduction in chronic opioid use—a prospective study		No
35047709	Croker	Medical cannabis and utilization of nonhospice palliative care services: complements and alternatives at end of life	https://doi.org/10.1093/geroni/igab048	No
35047242	Assanangkornchai	Medical cannabis use in Thailand after its legalization: a respondent-driven sample survey	https://doi.org/10.7717/peerj.12809	No
35040755	Caputi	The use of academic research in medical cannabis marketing: a qualitative and quantitative review of company websites		No
35030093	Diaz	Healing of a chronic pressure injury in a patient treated with medical cannabis for pain and sleep improvement: a case report		No
35025588	Berey	Differences in cannabis use characteristics, routines, and reasons for use among individuals with and without a medical cannabis card	https://doi.org/10.1037/pha0000542	No
35022250	Habib	Metabolic effects of medical cannabis treatment	https://doi.org/10.1136/jim-2021-002059	No
35012687	Thomas	Case report: medical cannabis-warfarin drug-drug interaction	https://doi.org/10.1186/s42238-021-00112-x	No
35009146	Crispim Massuela	Impact of harvest time and pruning technique on total CBD concentration and yield of medicinal cannabis	https://doi.org/10.3390/plants11010140	No
35005866	Yeroushalmi	Consumer perspectives on and utilization of medical cannabis to treat dermatologic conditions	https://doi.org/10.36849/JDD.2022.6540	No

(continued)

(continued)

PubMed ID	First author surname	Article title	DOI number	Citation included in the study (yes/no)
35004055	Balu	Medical cannabis certification is associated with decreased opiate use in patients with chronic pain: a retrospective cohort study in Delaware	https://doi.org/10.7759/cureus.20240	No
34999501	Edelstein	Attitudes and beliefs of medicine and social work students about medical cannabis use for epilepsy	https://doi.org/10.1016/j.yebeh.2021.108522	No
34999381	Caraballo	Long-term use of cannabidiol-enriched medical cannabis in a prospective cohort of children with drug-resistant developmental and epileptic encephalopathy	https://doi.org/10.1016/j.seizure.2022.01.001	No
34995571	Janatová	The chemical composition of ethanolic extracts from six genotypes of medical cannabis (*Cannabis sativa* L.) and their selective cytotoxic activity	https://doi.org/10.1016/j.cbi.2022.109800	No
34986005	Kitchen	Status and impacts of recreational and medicinal cannabis policies in Africa: a systematic review and thematic analysis of published and "gray" literature	https://doi.org/10.1089/can.2021.0110	No
34980282	Nimalan	UK medical cannabis registry palliative care patients cohort: initial experience and outcomes	https://doi.org/10.1186/s42238-021-00114-9	No
34940961	Tumati	Medical cannabis use among older adults in Canada: Self-reported data on types and amount used, and perceived effects	https://doi.org/10.1007/s40266-021-00913-y	No
34937477	Harris	UK medical cannabis registry: an analysis of clinical outcomes of medicinal cannabis therapy for chronic pain conditions	https://doi.org/10.1080/17512433.2022.2017771. Epub 2021 Dec 31	No
34937473	Ergisi	UK medical cannabis registry: an analysis of clinical outcomes of medicinal cannabis therapy for generalized anxiety disorder	https://doi.org/10.1080/17512433.2022.2020640	Yes
34930063	Bhagianadh	Legalization of medical cannabis and site of death: evidence from national vital statistics mortality data	https://doi.org/10.1177/07334648211058720	No

(continued)

(continued)

PubMed ID	First author surname	Article title	DOI number	Citation included in the study (yes/no)
34921662	Bonomo	Pharmacokinetics, safety, and tolerability of a medicinal cannabis formulation in patients with chronic non-cancer pain on long-term high dose opioid Analgesia: a pilot study	https://doi.org/10.1007/s40122-021-00344-y	No
34898143	Barata	Non-medical cannabis use: international policies and outcomes overview. An outline for Portugal	https://doi.org/10.47626/2237-6089-2021-0239	No
34893392	Fader	Assessment of medical cannabis in patients with osteoarthritis of the Thumb Basal joint	https://doi.org/10.1016/j.jhsa.2021.10.018	Yes—article was behind a paywall and could not be accessed
34893011	HaGani	Attitudes toward the use of medical cannabis and the perceived efficacy, side-effects and risks: a survey of patients, nurses and physicians	https://doi.org/10.1080/02791072.2021.2009598	Yes—Article was behind a paywall and could not be accessed
34887189	Bellnier	Description of collaborative, fee-for-service, office-based, pharmacist-directed medical cannabis therapy management service for patients with chronic pain	https://doi.org/10.1016/j.japh.2021.11.023	No
34874191	Siani-Rose	Cannabis-responsive biomarkers: a pharmacometabolomics-based application to evaluate the impact of medical cannabis treatment on children with autism spectrum disorder	https://doi.org/10.1089/can.2021.0129	No
37364019	Clobes	The impact of education on attitudes toward medical cannabis	https://doi.org/10.1016/j.pecinn.2021.100009	No
34844095	Hasin	Use of highly-potent cannabis concentrate products: more common in U.S. states with recreational or medical cannabis laws	https://doi.org/10.1016/j.drugalcdep.2021.109159	No
34843557	Landrum	Influences of study design on the effectiveness of consensus messaging: the case of medicinal cannabis	https://doi.org/10.1371/journal.pone.0260342	No
34828472	Russo	Innovative clinical-organizational model to ensure appropriateness and quality in the management of medical cannabis: an Italian regional case	https://doi.org/10.3390/healthcare9111425	No

(continued)

(continued)

PubMed ID	First author surname	Article title	DOI number	Citation included in the study (yes/no)
34821570	Tait	A quality-of-life evaluation study assessing health-related quality of life in patients receiving medicinal cannabis (the QUEST initiative): protocol for a longitudinal observational study	https://doi.org/10.2196/32327	No
34818602	Okey	Are recreational cannabis laws associated with declining medical cannabis program enrollment in the U.S.? An analysis of cardholder enrollment and demographic characteristics from 2013 to 2020	https://doi.org/10.1016/j.drugpo.2021.103531	No
34802466	Divisic	The use of medical cannabis in pediatric palliative care: a case series	https://doi.org/10.1186/s13052-021-01179-1	No
34802112	Petzke	Cannabis-based medicines and medical cannabis for chronic neuropathic pain	https://doi.org/10.1007/s40263-021-00879-w	No
34800285	Fitzcharles	Cannabis-based medicines and medical cannabis in the treatment of nociplastic pain	https://doi.org/10.1007/s40265-021-01602-1	No
34777039	Sznitman	Medical cannabis use and pain: an experience sampling study	https://doi.org/10.3389/fpsyt.2021.728283	No
34751862	Mauro	Medical and non-medical opioid use at the intersection of gender and sexual identity: associations with state medical cannabis law status in a U.S. national sample of adults	https://doi.org/10.1007/s10508-021-02128-z	No
34748204	Banerjee	Real world evidence in medical cannabis research	https://doi.org/10.1007/s43441-021-00346-0	No
34743399	Häuser	Register-based studies on cannabis-based medicines and medical cannabis need reliable diagnoses and cannabis treatment details	https://doi.org/10.1002/ejp.1881	No
34729274	Caputo	Medical cannabis as adjunctive therapy for head and neck cancer patients	https://doi.org/10.7759/cureus.18396	No

(continued)

(continued)

PubMed ID	First author surname	Article title	DOI number	Citation included in the study (yes/no)
34719005	Freckelton Ao Qc	Children as voices and images for medicinal cannabis law reform	https://doi.org/10.1007/s40592-021-00139-z	No
34715326	Isralowitz	CTIM editors' commentary: Special issue on medical cannabis in professional education	https://doi.org/10.1016/j.ctim.2021.102786	No
34695720	Goedel	Association of medical cannabis licensure with prescription opioid receipt: a population-based, individual-level retrospective cohort study	https://doi.org/10.1016/j.drugpo.2021.103502	No
34686558	Hallinan	Implementation of medicinal cannabis in Australia: innovation or upheaval? Perspectives from physicians as key informants, a qualitative analysis	https://doi.org/10.1136/bmjopen-2021-054044	Yes
34684842	Bennici	Safety of medical cannabis in neuropathic chronic pain management	https://doi.org/10.3390/molecules26206257	No
34676351	Brown	Evidence in context: high risk of bias in medical cannabis and cannabinoid clinical trials dictates the need for cautious interpretation	https://doi.org/10.1159/000514732	No
34676348	Jugl	A mapping literature review of medical cannabis clinical outcomes and quality of evidence in approved conditions in the USA from 2016 to 2019	https://doi.org/10.1159/000515069	No
34674661	Rønne	Physicians' experiences, attitudes, and beliefs towards medical cannabis: a systematic literature review	https://doi.org/10.1186/s12875-021-01559-w	Yes
34671723	Wang	Health outcomes among adults initiating medical cannabis for chronic pain: a 3-month prospective study incorporating ecological momentary assessment (EMA)	https://doi.org/10.26828/cannabis/2021.02.006	No
34664109	Peters	Pharmacokinetics of cannabichromene in a medical cannabis product also containing cannabidiol and Δ(9)-tetrahydrocannabinol: a pilot study	https://doi.org/10.1007/s00228-021-03232-8	No

(continued)

(continued)

PubMed ID	First author surname	Article title	DOI number	Citation included in the study (yes/no)
34663604	Huntsman	Improving the regulation of medical cannabis in Canada to better serve pediatric patients	https://doi.org/10.1503/cmaj.202169	No
34649577	Ruheel	Facilitators and barriers to the regulation of medical cannabis: a scoping review of the peer-reviewed literature	https://doi.org/10.1186/s12954-021-00547-8	No
34646751	Anderson Goodell	Feasibility and acceptability of using smartphone-based EMA to assess patterns of prescription opioid and medical cannabis use among individuals with chronic pain	https://doi.org/10.1016/j.invent.2021.100460	No
34645786	Poleg	Behavioral aspects and neurobiological properties underlying medical cannabis treatment in Shank3 mouse model of autism spectrum disorder	https://doi.org/10.1038/s41398-021-01612-3	No
34641976	Weisman	A systematic review of medical students' and professionals' attitudes and knowledge regarding medical cannabis	https://doi.org/10.1186/s42238-021-00100-1	No
34640561	Hordowicz	Polish physicians' perspectives on medical cannabis policy and educational needs: results of an online survey	https://doi.org/10.3390/jcm10194545	Yes
34631734	Zaiachuk	Cannabinoids, medical cannabis, and colorectal cancer immunotherapy	https://doi.org/10.3389/fmed.2021.713153	No
34628531	Duarte	Medical cannabis for headache pain: a primer for clinicians	https://doi.org/10.1007/s11916-021-00974-z	No
34624613	Caraballo	Cannabidiol-enriched medical cannabis as add-on therapy in children with treatment-resistant West syndrome: a study of eight patients	https://doi.org/10.1016/j.seizure.2021.10.002	Yes
34624164	Hjorthøj	Cannabis-based medicines and medical cannabis for patients with neuropathic pain and other pain disorders: nationwide register-based pharmacoepidemiologic comparison with propensity score matched controls	https://doi.org/10.1002/ejp.1874	No
34607636	Perlman	Medical cannabis state and federal regulations: implications for United States health care entities	https://doi.org/10.1016/j.mayocp.2021.05.005	No

(continued)

(continued)

PubMed ID	First author surname	Article title	DOI number	Citation included in the study (yes/no)
34593176	Erku	Cost-effectiveness of medicinal cannabis for management of refractory symptoms associated with chronic conditions: a systematic review of economic evaluations	https://doi.org/10.1016/j.jval.2021.04.1276	No
37287530	Sagar	Assessing cannabis use disorder in medical cannabis patients: interim analyses from an observational, longitudinal study	https://doi.org/10.26828/cannabis/2021.02.004	No
34590094	Henderson	Medicinal cannabis in the treatment of chronic pain	https://doi.org/10.31128/AJGP-04-21-5939	No
34589318	Poudel	Medical cannabis, headaches, and migraines: a review of the current literature	https://doi.org/10.7759/cureus.17407	No
34587580	Kim	Association between fatal opioid overdose and state medical cannabis laws in US national survey data, 2000–2011	https://doi.org/10.1016/j.drugpo.2021.103449	No
34579367	Danziger	Shape matters: plant architecture affects chemical uniformity in large-size medical cannabis plants	https://doi.org/10.3390/plants10091834	No
34570205	Martins	Racial and ethnic differences in cannabis use following legalization in US States with medical cannabis laws	https://doi.org/10.1001/jamanetworkopen.2021.27002	No
34567876	Khurshid	A systematic review of fibromyalgia and recent advancements in treatment: is medicinal cannabis a new hope?	https://doi.org/10.7759/cureus.17332	No
34566726	Martin	Antidepressant and anxiolytic effects of medicinal cannabis use in an observational trial	https://doi.org/10.3389/fpsyt.2021.729800	No
34562980	Lowe	The current and potential application of medicinal cannabis products in dentistry	https://doi.org/10.3390/dj9090106	No
34551006	Matchett-Oates	In silico analysis enabling informed design for genome editing in medicinal cannabis; gene families and variant characterisation	https://doi.org/10.1371/journal.pone.0257413	No
34546363	AminiLari	Medical cannabis and cannabinoids for impaired sleep: a systematic review and meta-analysis of randomized clinical trials	https://doi.org/10.1093/sleep/zsab234	Yes

(continued)

(continued)

PubMed ID	First author surname	Article title	DOI number	Citation included in the study (yes/no)
34538843	Aviram	Sex differences in medical cannabis-related adverse effects	https://doi.org/10.1097/j.pain.0000000000002463	No
34531934	Habib	The effect of medical cannabis on pain level and quality of sleep among rheumatology clinic outpatients	https://doi.org/10.1155/2021/1756588	No
34524435	Merlin	Analysis of state cannabis laws and dispensary staff recommendations to adults purchasing medical cannabis	https://doi.org/10.1001/jamanetworkopen.2021.24511	No
34521640	Sznitman	Opioid and healthcare service use in medical cannabis patients with chronic pain: a prospective study	https://doi.org/10.1136/bmjspcare-2020-002661	No
34507536	Zongo	Medical cannabis authorization and the risk of cardiovascular events: a longitudinal cohort study	https://doi.org/10.1186/s12872-021-02229-6	No
34497094	Kröger	Medical cannabis for chronic pain	https://doi.org/10.1136/bmj.n1942	No
34497062	Busse	Medical cannabis or cannabinoids for chronic pain: a clinical practice guideline	https://doi.org/10.1136/bmj.n2040	No
34497049	Mahase	Offer medical cannabis to patients with chronic pain, experts recommend	https://doi.org/10.1136/bmj.n2208	No
34497047	Wang	Medical cannabis or cannabinoids for chronic non-cancer and cancer related pain: a systematic review and meta-analysis of randomised clinical trials	https://doi.org/10.1136/bmj.n1034	No
34493521	Zeng	Values and preferences towards medical cannabis among people living with chronic pain: a mixed-methods systematic review	https://doi.org/10.1136/bmjopen-2021-050831	No
34479659	Neben-Wittich	Medical cannabis to treat symptoms from head and neck radiation therapy	https://doi.org/10.1016/j.prro.2021.03.007	No
34476478	Adler	Primary care physicians' attitudes and knowledge regarding medical cannabis and willingness to prescribe it: the Israeli experience	https://doi.org/10.1093/fampra/cmab108	Yes

(continued)

(continued)

PubMed ID	First author surname	Article title	DOI number	Citation included in the study (yes/no)
34473850	Kawka	Clinical outcome data of first cohort of chronic pain patients treated with cannabis-based sublingual oils in the United Kingdom: analysis from the UK medical cannabis registry	https://doi.org/10.1002/jcph.1961	No
34465496	Fischer	Lower-risk cannabis use guidelines (LRCUG) for reducing health harms from non-medical cannabis use: a comprehensive evidence and recommendations update	https://doi.org/10.1016/j.drugpo.2021.103381	No
34463161	Kruger	Assessing health care providers' knowledge of medical cannabis	https://doi.org/10.1089/can.2021.0032	No
34432543	Holdman	Safety and efficacy of medical cannabis in autism spectrum disorder compared with commonly used medications	https://doi.org/10.1089/can.2020.0154	Yes
34425501	Kudahl	Medical cannabis and cannabis-based medicine show both potential efficacy and potential harms: cross-sectional comparison with controls on self-rated and interviewer-rated outcomes within the Danish pilot program on medical cannabis	https://doi.org/10.1016/j.ctcp.2021.101476	No
34411246	Ross	First-year trajectories of medical cannabis use among adults taking opioids for chronic pain: an observational cohort study	https://doi.org/10.1093/pm/pnab257	No
34403168	Fletcher	Medicinal cannabis in children and adolescents with autism spectrum disorder: a scoping review	https://doi.org/10.1111/cch.12909	Yes
34350559	Clarke	In reply: comment on: patient-reported outcomes in those consuming medical cannabis: a prospective longitudinal observational study in patients with chronic pain	https://doi.org/10.1007/s12630-021-02079-y	No
34350557	Vitetta	Comment on: patient-reported outcomes in those consuming medical cannabis: a prospective longitudinal observational study in patients with chronic pain	https://doi.org/10.1007/s12630-021-02078-z	No
34335641	Shiponi	The highs and lows of p supply in medical cannabis: effects on cannabinoids, the ionome, and morpho-physiology	https://doi.org/10.3389/fpls.2021.657323	No

(continued)

(continued)

PubMed ID	First author surname	Article title	DOI number	Citation included in the study (yes/no)
34321302	Noori	Opioid-sparing effects of medical cannabis or cannabinoids for chronic pain: a systematic review and meta-analysis of randomised and observational studies	https://doi.org/10.1136/bmjopen-2020-047717	No
34321108	Lucas	The impact of non-medical cannabis legalization and other exposures on retention in longitudinal cannabis research: a survival analysis of a prospective study of Canadian medical cannabis patients	https://doi.org/10.1186/s42238-021-00089-7	No
34309706	Zürcher	Use and caregiver-reported efficacy of medical cannabis in children and adolescents in Switzerland	https://doi.org/10.1007/s00431-021-04202-z	No
34301703	Dar	Treating pain related to Ehlers-Danlos syndrome with medical cannabis	https://doi.org/10.1136/bcr-2021-242568	No
34281626	Lazarjani	Processing and extraction methods of medicinal cannabis: a narrative review	https://doi.org/10.1186/s42238-021-00087-9	No
34261553	Sagar	An observational, longitudinal study of cognition in medical cannabis patients over the course of 12 months of treatment: preliminary results	https://doi.org/10.1017/S1355617721000114	No
34258798	Lebesmuehlbacher	The effect of medical cannabis laws on pharmaceutical marketing to physicians	https://doi.org/10.1002/hec.4380	No
34252785	Qatanani	Bioethical insights from the Fiqh Council of North America's recent ruling on medical cannabis	https://doi.org/10.1016/j.drugpo.2021.103360	No
34252784	Gunning	Coverage of medical cannabis by Canadian news media: ethics, access, and policy	https://doi.org/10.1016/j.drugpo.2021.103361	No
34240307	Smith	An exploration of self-reported medicinal cannabis use among a sample of Eastern Canadian postsecondary students	https://doi.org/10.1007/s11414-021-09763-3	No
34234177	Jerushalmi	Effects of steam sterilization on reduction of fungal colony forming units, cannabinoids and terpene levels in medical cannabis inflorescences	https://doi.org/10.1038/s41598-021-93264-y	No

(continued)

(continued)

PubMed ID	First author surname	Article title	DOI number	Citation included in the study (yes/no)
34232478	Jouanjus	Establishing and evaluating a study questionnaire on knowledge and attitudes of healthcare professionals towards recreational and medical cannabis across Europe	https://doi.org/10.1007/s40261-021-01058-x	No
34225825	Orjuela-Rojas	Medicinal cannabis: knowledge, beliefs, and attitudes of Colombian psychiatrists	https://doi.org/10.1186/s42238-021-00083-z	Yes
34215346	Bhaskar	Consensus recommendations on dosing and administration of medical cannabis to treat chronic pain: results of a modified Delphi process	https://doi.org/10.1186/s42238-021-00073-1	No
34214413	O'Connell	Trends in cannabis-related attitudes and behaviors among cannabis-using adolescent and young adult outpatients following medical cannabis legalization in Massachusetts	https://doi.org/10.1080/08897077.2021.1941517	No
34190709	Shastay	As approval of medical cannabis spreads state by state, product Labeling improvements are a must	https://doi.org/10.1097/NHH.0000000000000992	No
34174826	Naim-Feil	The characterization of key physiological traits of medicinal cannabis (*Cannabis sativa* L.) as a tool for precision breeding	https://doi.org/10.1186/s12870-021-03079-2	No
34162446	Rapin	Cannabidiol use and effectiveness: real-world evidence from a Canadian medical cannabis clinic	https://doi.org/10.1186/s42238-021-00078-w	No
34155769	Philip	Fact versus fiction: bridging contrasting medicinal cannabis information needs	https://doi.org/10.1111/imj.15361	No
34155601	Taylor	Factors associated with cannabis use during the reproductive cycle: a retrospective cross-sectional study of women in states with recreational and medical cannabis legalization	https://doi.org/10.1007/s10995-021-03197-1	No
34139340	Bonnici	Maltese health and social wellbeing student knowledge, attitudes and beliefs about medical cannabis	https://doi.org/10.1016/j.ctim.2021.102753	No

(continued)

(continued)

PubMed ID	First author surname	Article title	DOI number	Citation included in the study (yes/no)
34118713	Lucas	Self-reported reductions in tobacco and nicotine use following medical cannabis initiation: results from a cross-sectional survey of authorized medical cannabis patients in Canada	https://doi.org/10.1016/j.jsat.2021.108481	No
34115851	Walsh	Treating insomnia symptoms with medicinal cannabis: a randomized, crossover trial of the efficacy of a cannabinoid medicine compared with placebo	https://doi.org/10.1093/sleep/zsab149	Yes
34107448	Perkins	Medicinal cannabis and driving: the intersection of health and road safety policy	https://doi.org/10.1016/j.drugpo.2021.103307	No
34095048	Cahill	Evaluation of patient reported safety and efficacy of cannabis from a survey of medical cannabis patients in Canada	https://doi.org/10.3389/fpubh.2021.626853	No
34094937	Schloss	A phase 2 randomised clinical trial assessing the tolerability of two different ratios of medicinal cannabis in patients with high grade gliomas	https://doi.org/10.3389/fonc.2021.649555	No
34093173	Aviram	Prolonged medical cannabis treatment is associated with quality of life improvement and reduction of analgesic medication consumption in chronic pain patients	https://doi.org/10.3389/fphar.2021.613805	No
34085149	Zylla	A randomized trial of medical cannabis in patients with stage IV cancers to assess feasibility, dose requirements, impact on pain and opioid use, safety, and overall patient satisfaction	https://doi.org/10.1007/s00520-021-06301-x	No
34083092	MacCallum	"Is medical cannabis safe for my patients?" A practical review of cannabis safety considerations	https://doi.org/10.1016/j.ejim.2021.05.002	No
34071473	Qamar	Development and optimization of supercritical fluid extraction setup leading to quantification of 11 cannabinoids derived from medicinal cannabis	https://doi.org/10.3390/biology10060481	No
34059839	Herbert	Medicinal cannabis use in palliative care	https://doi.org/10.31128/AJGP-02-21-5831	No

(continued)

(continued)

PubMed ID	First author surname	Article title	DOI number	Citation included in the study (yes/no)
34059837	Arnold	A primer on medicinal cannabis safety and potential adverse effects	https://doi.org/10.31128/AJGP-02-21-5845	No
34059836	Arkell	Medical cannabis and driving	https://doi.org/10.31128/AJGP-02-21-5840	No
34059835	Duns	Editorial: Medical cannabis—progress and promise	https://doi.org/10.31128/AJGP-06-21-1234e	No
34052339	Prosk	The model of care at a leading medical cannabis clinic in Canada	https://doi.org/10.1016/j.ctim.2021.102740	No
34044878	Mahabir	Comparing medical cannabis use in 5 US states: a retrospective database study	https://doi.org/10.1186/s42238-021-00075-z	No
34044753	Fedorova	Changes in medical cannabis patient status before and after cannabis legalization in california: associations with cannabis and other drug use	https://doi.org/10.1080/02791072.2021.1926604	No
34021014	Gibbard	Family attitudes about and experiences with medical cannabis in children with cancer or epilepsy: an exploratory qualitative study	https://doi.org/10.9778/cmajo.20200212	No
34002633	Croker	Cannabis and end-of-life care: a snapshot of hospice planning and experiences among Illinois medical cannabis patients with a terminal diagnosis	https://doi.org/10.1177/10499091211018655	No
34000362	Aviram	Specific phytocannabinoid compositions are associated with analgesic response and adverse effects in chronic pain patients treated with medical cannabis	https://doi.org/10.1016/j.phrs.2021.105651	No
33999649	Kalaba	Cannabinoid profiles in medical cannabis users: effects of age, gender, symptoms, and duration of use	https://doi.org/10.1089/can.2020.0120	No
33998902	Kalaba	Authorization patterns, safety, and effectiveness of medical cannabis in Quebec	https://doi.org/10.1089/can.2020.0140	No
33998897	Shulman	Evolving global perspectives of pharmacists: dispensing medical cannabis	https://doi.org/10.1089/can.2020.0144	No

(continued)

(continued)

PubMed ID	First author surname	Article title	DOI number	Citation included in the study (yes/no)
33998878	El-Khoury	Legalizing medical cannabis in Lebanon: the complex interface between medicine, law, ethics, and economics	https://doi.org/10.1089/can.2020.0108	No
33998868	Kaufmann	Patterns of medical cannabis use among older adults from a cannabis dispensary in New York State	https://doi.org/10.1089/can.2020.0064	No
33998852	Schlienz	A cross-sectional and prospective comparison of medicinal cannabis users and controls on self-reported health	https://doi.org/10.1089/can.2019.0096	No
33995035	MacCallum	Practical strategies using medical cannabis to reduce harms associated with long term opioid use in chronic pain	https://doi.org/10.3389/fphar.2021.633168	No
33988306	Erridge	An initial analysis of the UK medical cannabis registry: outcomes analysis of first 129 patients	https://doi.org/10.1002/npr2.12183	No
33956129	Matson	Prevalence of medical cannabis use and associated health conditions documented in electronic health records among primary care patients in Washington State	https://doi.org/10.1001/jamanetworkopen.2021.9375	No
33955716	Sannes	United States oncologists' clinical preferences regarding modes of medicinal cannabis use	https://doi.org/10.1002/cac2.12160	No
33940011	Schlag	Current controversies in medical cannabis: recent developments in human clinical applications and potential therapeutics	https://doi.org/10.1016/j.neuropharm.2021.108586	No
33938797	Fitzcharles	Use of medical cannabis by patients with fibromyalgia in Canada after cannabis legalisation: a cross-sectional study	https://doi.org/10.55563/clinexprheumatol/qcyet7	No
33933061	Lee	Opioid use in medical cannabis authorization adult patients from 2013 to 2018: Alberta, Canada	https://doi.org/10.1186/s12889-021-10867-w	No
33932156	Chapman	Medical cannabis in pediatric oncology: a survey of patients and caregivers	https://doi.org/10.1007/s00520-021-06202-z	No
33930337	Saffier	Medicinal cannabis: new challenges for the anesthesiologist	https://doi.org/10.1016/j.bjane.2021.02.056	No

(continued)

(continued)

PubMed ID	First author surname	Article title	DOI number	Citation included in the study (yes/no)
33927439	Rychert	Predictors of medicinal cannabis users' willingness to utilise a new prescription Medicinal Cannabis Scheme in New Zealand		No
33915068	Choi	Comparing older nonmedical and medical cannabis users: health-related characteristics, cannabis use patterns, and cannabis sources	https://doi.org/10.1080/00952990.2021.1908318	No
33911061		Medical Cannabis	https://doi.org/10.1097/NJH.0000000000000751	No
33908299	Hall	Easier patient access to medical cannabis carries risks as well as benefits	https://doi.org/10.1177/02698811211009798	No
33906699	Lee	Cohort study of medical cannabis authorization and motor vehicle crash-related healthcare visits in 2014–2017 in Ontario, Canada	https://doi.org/10.1186/s40621-021-00321-1	No
33897066	Urits	Adverse effects of recreational and medical cannabis		No
33864906	Likhitsathian	Cross national comparison of medical students' attitudes and beliefs about medical cannabis and its application for pain management	https://doi.org/10.1016/j.ctim.2021.102720	No
33849983	Ng	Attitudes toward medical cannabis among family physicians practising in Ontario, Canada: a qualitative research study	https://doi.org/10.9778/cmajo.20200187	Yes
33848611	Bai	Archaeobotanical evidence of the use of medicinal cannabis in a secular context unearthed from south China	https://doi.org/10.1016/j.jep.2021.114114	No
33847549	Zhou	Cancer patient's attitudes of using medicinal cannabis for sleep	https://doi.org/10.1080/07347332.2021.1910396	No
33844003	Gilman	Variation in cannabinoid metabolites present in the urine of adults using medical cannabis products in Massachusetts	https://doi.org/10.1001/jamanetworkopen.2021.5490	No
33812039	Findle	Attitudes and beliefs about medical cannabis among social work students: cross-national comparison	https://doi.org/10.1016/j.ctim.2021.102716	No

(continued)

(continued)

PubMed ID	First author surname	Article title	DOI number	Citation included in the study (yes/no)
33795939	Vannabouathong	Can medical cannabis therapies be cost-effective in the non-surgical management of chronic knee pain?	https://doi.org/10.1177/117954412110 02492	No
33794932	Rychert	Foreign investment in emerging legal medicinal cannabis markets: the Jamaica case study	https://doi.org/10.1186/s12 992-021-006 87-3	No
33790818	Eadie	Duration of neurocognitive impairment with medical cannabis use: a scoping review	https://doi.org/10.3389/fpsyt. 2021.638962	No
33765514	Richard	How medical are states' medical cannabis policies?: Proposing a standardized scale	https://doi.org/10.1016/j.dru gpo.2021. 103202	No
33764103	Gruber	No pain, all gain? Interim analyses from a longitudinal, observational study examining the impact of medical cannabis treatment on chronic pain and related symptoms	https://doi.org/10.1037/pha 0000435	No
33747008	Adhikary	Medical Cannabis and industrial hemp tissue culture: present status and future potential	https://doi.org/10.3389/fpls. 2021.627240	No
33735318	DiDiodato	Elicitation of stakeholder viewpoints about medical cannabis research for pain management in critically ill ventilated patients: a Q-methodology study	https://doi.org/10.1371/jou rnal.pone.024 8475	No
33726006	Shaffer	Application of medical cannabis in unstable angina and coronary artery disease: a case report	https://doi.org/10.1097/MD. 000000000002 5172	No
33725004	Cousins	Differences between cancer patients and others who use medicinal Cannabis	https://doi.org/10.1371/jou rnal.pone.024 8227	No
33716092	Isralowitz	Toward medical cannabis education in Israel	https://doi.org/10.1016/j.ctim. 2021.102709	No
33677020	Felnhofer	Knowledge about and attitudes towards medical cannabis among Austrian university students	https://doi.org/10.1016/j.ctim. 2021.102700	No
33675934	Sokratous	Medical cannabis attitudes, beliefs and knowledge among Greek-Cypriot University nursing students	https://doi.org/10.1016/j.ctim. 2021.102707	No

(continued)

(continued)

PubMed ID	First author surname	Article title	DOI number	Citation included in the study (yes/no)
33671711	Konstantinov	Foreign medical students in Eastern Europe: knowledge, attitudes and beliefs about medical cannabis for pain management	https://doi.org/10.3390/ijerph18042137	No
33664541		More prescribing resources for medicinal cannabis	https://doi.org/10.18773/austprescr.2020.085	No
33647397	Giannakopoulou	Attitudes, beliefs and knowledge towards medical cannabis of Greek undergraduate and postgraduate university nursing students	https://doi.org/10.1016/j.ctim.2021.102703	No
33636612	Guarnaccia	Patterns of medical cannabis use among patients diagnosed with multiple sclerosis	https://doi.org/10.1016/j.msard.2021.102830	Yes—article was behind a paywall and could not be accessed
33621991	Kaufman	Opioid mortality following implementation of medical cannabis programs in the United States	https://doi.org/10.1055/a-1353-6509	No
33614954	Reece	Survey of pharmacists' knowledge of connecticut's medical cannabis program	https://doi.org/10.1089/can.2019.0013	Yes
33613794	Chang	Medical cannabis for chronic noncancer pain: a systematic review of health care recommendations	https://doi.org/10.1155/2021/8857948	No
33597032	Mazza	Medical cannabis for the treatment of fibromyalgia syndrome: a retrospective, open-label case series	https://doi.org/10.1186/s42238-021-00060-6	No
33577600	Habib	The impact of medical cannabis consumption on the oral flora and saliva	https://doi.org/10.1371/journal.pone.0247044	No
33571928	Zolotov	Attitudes and knowledge about medical cannabis among Israeli and American nursing students	https://doi.org/10.1016/j.nedt.2021.104789	No
33567970	Ryan	Medicinal cannabis: policy, patients, and providers	https://doi.org/10.1177/1527154421989609	No
33565655	Mair	Availability of medical cannabis dispensaries and cannabis abuse/dependence-related hospitalizations in California	https://doi.org/10.1111/add.15420	No

(continued)

(continued)

PubMed ID	First author surname	Article title	DOI number	Citation included in the study (yes/no)
33539943	Zolotov	Medical cannabis education among healthcare trainees: a scoping review	https://doi.org/10.1016/j.ctim.2021.102675	No
33526141	Wyse	Trends in intellectual property rights protection for medical cannabis and related products	https://doi.org/10.1186/s42238-020-00057-7	No
33526140	Boehnke	Communication between healthcare providers and medical cannabis patients regarding referral and medication substitution	https://doi.org/10.1186/s42238-021-00058-0	No
33526139	Aliekperova	Perspectives on formation of medical cannabis market in Ukraine based on holistic approach	https://doi.org/10.1186/s42238-020-00044-y	No
33526127	Kruger	A content analysis of internet information sources on medical cannabis	https://doi.org/10.1186/s42238-020-00041-1	No
33526119	Ben-Ishay	Smokeless consumption of medical cannabis pharmacokinetics, safety and feasibility of the CannaHALER© a phase 1a study	https://doi.org/10.1186/s42238-020-00022-4	No
33526115	Lombardi	Ohio physician attitudes toward medical Cannabis and Ohio's medical marijuana program	https://doi.org/10.1186/s42238-020-00025-1	No
33526110	Mahabir	Medical cannabis use in the United States: a retrospective database study	https://doi.org/10.1186/s42238-020-00038-w	No
33526086	Jerushalmi	Effects of cold plasma, gamma and e-beam irradiations on reduction of fungal colony forming unit levels in medical cannabis inflorescences	https://doi.org/10.1186/s42238-020-00020-6	No
33517127	Caputi	What cannabis can learn from Covid: hydroxychloroquine research suggests the next step for medical cannabis research	https://doi.org/10.1016/j.drugpo.2021.103133	No
33503640	Koslowsky	Gastroenterologists' attitude regarding medical cannabis for inflammatory bowel diseases in Israel	https://doi.org/10.1159/000514776	No
33494156	Arias	Clinical evidence of Magistral preparations based on medicinal cannabis	https://doi.org/10.3390/ph14020078	No

(continued)

(continued)

PubMed ID	First author surname	Article title	DOI number	Citation included in the study (yes/no)
33486047	Khamenka	Knowledge, attitudes and beliefs about medical cannabis among the medical students of the Belarus State Medical University	https://doi.org/10.1016/j.ctim.2021.102670	No
33469735	Meng	Patient-reported outcomes in those consuming medical cannabis: a prospective longitudinal observational study in chronic pain patients	https://doi.org/10.1007/s12630-020-01903-1	No
33460744	Luque	Mixed methods study of the potential therapeutic benefits from medical cannabis for patients in Florida	https://doi.org/10.1016/j.ctim.2021.102669	No
33451073	Busardò	Disposition of phytocannabinoids, their acidic precursors and their metabolites in biological matrices of healthy individuals treated with vaporized medical cannabis	https://doi.org/10.3390/ph14010059	No
33439370	Abu-Amna	Medical cannabis in oncology: a valuable unappreciated remedy or an undesirable risk?	https://doi.org/10.1007/s11864-020-00811-2	No
33416237	Abo Ziad	The attitudes and beliefs of family physicians regarding the use of medical cannabis, knowledge of side effects, and barriers to use: a comparison between residents and specialists	https://doi.org/10.1097/MJT.0000000000001236	Yes—article was behind a paywall and could not be accessed
33413454	McGinty	Protocol: mixed-methods study of how implementation of US state medical cannabis laws affects treatment of chronic non-cancer pain and adverse opioid outcomes	https://doi.org/10.1186/s13012-020-01071-2	No
33409086	Takakuwa	A survey on the effect that medical cannabis has on prescription opioid medication usage for the treatment of chronic pain at three medical cannabis practice sites	https://doi.org/10.7759/cureus.11848	No
33404120	Monaghan	Scandalous decisions: explaining shifts in UK medicinal cannabis policy	https://doi.org/10.1111/add.15350	No
33400332	Coughlin	Progression of cannabis withdrawal symptoms in people using medical cannabis for chronic pain	https://doi.org/10.1111/add.15370	No

(continued)

(continued)

PubMed ID	First author surname	Article title	DOI number	Citation included in the study (yes/no)
33387864		Safety and efficacy of low-dose medical cannabis oils in multiple sclerosis	https://doi.org/10.1016/j.msard.2020.102708	Yes—article was behind a paywall and could not be accessed
33376181	Cunningham	Medical Marijuana and Opioids (MEMO) Study: protocol of a longitudinal cohort study to examine if medical cannabis reduces opioid use among adults with chronic pain	https://doi.org/10.1136/bmjopen-2020-043400	No
33364946	Dei Cas	Phytocannabinoids profile in medicinal cannabis oils: the impact of plant varieties and preparation methods	https://doi.org/10.3389/fphar.2020.570616	No
33360735	Wennberg	Non-medical cannabis use among Indigenous Canadians: a systematic review of prevalence and associated factors	https://doi.org/10.1016/j.drugpo.2020.103081	No
33353993		Erratum: prescribing medicinal cannabis [correction]	https://doi.org/10.18773/austprescr.2020.073	No
33343771	Parihar	Mandatory pharmacist-led education session for patients seeking medical cannabis	https://doi.org/10.18549/PharmPract.2020.4.2088	No
33337931	Kurlyandchik	Safety and efficacy of medicinal cannabis in the treatment of fibromyalgia: a systematic review	https://doi.org/10.1089/acm.2020.0331	Yes—article was behind a paywall and could not be accessed
33328530	Linciano	Identification of a new cannabidiol n-hexyl homolog in a medicinal cannabis variety with an antinociceptive activity in mice: cannabidihexol	https://doi.org/10.1038/s41598-020-79042-2	No
33322849	Pérez-Acevedo	Disposition of cannabidiol metabolites in serum and urine from healthy individuals treated with pharmaceutical preparations of medical cannabis	https://doi.org/10.3390/ph13120459	No
33312185	Saloner	Response of medical cannabis (*Cannabis sativa* L.) to nitrogen supply under long photoperiod	https://doi.org/10.3389/fpls.2020.572293	No
33307207	Temple	CTIM editors' commentary: special issue on medical cannabis	https://doi.org/10.1016/j.ctim.2020.102641	No
33298281	Pichini	UHPLC-MS/MS analysis of cannabidiol metabolites in serum and urine samples. Application to an individual treated with medical cannabis	https://doi.org/10.1016/j.talanta.2020.121772	No

(continued)

(continued)

PubMed ID	First author surname	Article title	DOI number	Citation included in the study (yes/no)
33283285	Wagner	From community of practice to epistemic community—law, discipline and security in the battle for the legalisation of medical cannabis in Poland	https://doi.org/10.1111/1467-9566.13217	No
33265945	Aviram	Short-term medical cannabis treatment regimens produced beneficial effects among palliative cancer patients	https://doi.org/10.3390/ph13120435	No
33256496	Hergert	Use of medical cannabis to treat traumatic brain injury	https://doi.org/10.1089/neu.2020.7148	Yes
33250007	Manning	Medical cannabis use: exploring the perceptions and experiences of older adults with chronic conditions	https://doi.org/10.1080/07317115.2020.1853299	Yes—article was behind a paywall and could not be accessed
33220620	Yeroushalmi	Perceptions and recommendation behaviors of dermatologists for medical cannabis: a pilot survey	https://doi.org/10.1016/j.ctim.2020.102552	No
33215230	Gressler	Exploring the use of state medical cannabis legislation as a proxy for medical cannabis use among patients receiving chemotherapy	https://doi.org/10.1007/s11864-020-00803-2	No
33213975	Carnide	Patterns and correlates of workplace and non-workplace cannabis use among Canadian workers before the legalization of non-medical cannabis	https://doi.org/10.1016/j.drugalcdep.2020.108386	No
33208249	Cox	Implications of the 2018 Canadian cannabis act: should regulation differ for medicinal and non-medicinal cannabis use?	https://doi.org/10.1016/j.healthpol.2020.10.016	No
33204797	Webster	Prescribed medical cannabis in women with gynecologic malignancies: a single-institution survey-based study	https://doi.org/10.1016/j.gore.2020.100667	No
33197667	Zolotov	Preliminary assessment of medical cannabis consumption by cancer survivors	https://doi.org/10.1016/j.ctim.2020.102592	No
33183664	Gritsenko	Religion in Russia: its impact on university student medical cannabis attitudes and beliefs	https://doi.org/10.1016/j.ctim.2020.102546	No
33165173	Fletcher	Symptoms, adverse events, and outcomes in the use of medicinal cannabis in children and adolescents with autism spectrum disorder: a scoping review protocol	https://doi.org/10.11124/JBIES-20-00001	No

(continued)

(continued)

PubMed ID	First author surname	Article title	DOI number	Citation included in the study (yes/no)
33155722	Pérez-Acevedo	Disposition of cannabinoids and their metabolites in serum, oral fluid, sweat patch and urine from healthy individuals treated with pharmaceutical preparations of medical cannabis	https://doi.org/10.1002/ptr.6931	No
33151533	Philbrick	Education and attitudes on medical cannabis in family medicine residency programs	https://doi.org/10.22454/FamMed.2020.645274	No
33093741	Arnold	Prescribing medicinal cannabis	https://doi.org/10.18773/austprescr.2020.052	No
33093301	Davidson	Anesthetic considerations in medical cannabis patients	https://doi.org/10.1097/ACO.0000000000000932	No
33090932	Bruce	Gender differences in medical cannabis use: symptoms treated, physician support for use, and prescription medication discontinuation	https://doi.org/10.1089/jwh.2020.8437	No
33073397	Shakeri	The missed opportunity for real-world evidence to shape our understanding of medical cannabis	https://doi.org/10.1111/bcp.14550	No
33068830	Lucas	Reductions in alcohol use following medical cannabis initiation: results from a large cross-sectional survey of medical cannabis patients in Canada	https://doi.org/10.1016/j.drugpo.2020.102963	No
33065768	Aviram	Medical cannabis treatment for chronic pain: outcomes and prediction of response	https://doi.org/10.1002/ejp.1675	No
33017729	Arkell	Driving-related behaviours, attitudes and perceptions among Australian medical cannabis users: results from the CAMS 18–19 Survey	https://doi.org/10.1016/j.aap.2020.105784	No
33009244	Zinboonyahgoon	Medicinal cannabis in Thailand: 1-year experience after legalization	https://doi.org/10.1097/j.pain.0000000000001936	No
32986266	Braun	Cancer patients' experiences with medicinal cannabis-related care	https://doi.org/10.1002/cncr.33202	No
32964502	Sznitman	Medical cannabis and cognitive performance in middle to old adults treated for chronic pain	https://doi.org/10.1111/dar.13171	No

(continued)

(continued)

PubMed ID	First author surname	Article title	DOI number	Citation included in the study (yes/no)
32958492	Nutt	So near yet so far: why won't the UK prescribe medical cannabis?	https://doi.org/10.1136/bmjopen-2020-038687	No
32924552	Kogan	Medical cannabis: a new old tool for palliative care	https://doi.org/10.1089/acm.2019.0184	No
32923663	Takakuwa	The impact of medical cannabis on intermittent and chronic opioid users with back pain: how cannabis diminished prescription opioid usage	https://doi.org/10.1089/can.2019.0039	No
32923659	Reimann-Philipp	Cannabis Chemovar nomenclature misrepresents chemical and genetic diversity; survey of variations in chemical profiles and genetic markers in Nevada medical cannabis samples	https://doi.org/10.1089/can.2018.0063	No
32919002	Öblom	Data-enriched edible pharmaceuticals (DEEP) of medical cannabis by inkjet printing	https://doi.org/10.1016/j.ijpharm.2020.119866	No
32906770	Pichini	Medicinal cannabis and synthetic cannabinoid use	https://doi.org/10.3390/medicina56090453	No
32892960	Mostafavi	Autism spectrum disorder and medical cannabis: review and clinical experience	https://doi.org/10.1016/j.spen.2020.100833	No
32889833	Macari	Medical cannabis in cancer patients: a survey of a community hematology oncology population	https://doi.org/10.1097/COC.0000000000000718	No
32887067	Berman	Cannabinoidomics—an analytical approach to understand the effect of medical cannabis treatment on the endocannabinoid metabolome	https://doi.org/10.1016/j.talanta.2020.121336	No
32842935	Croker	Assessing health-related outcomes of medical cannabis use among older persons: findings from Colorado and Illinois	https://doi.org/10.1080/07317115.2020.1797971	No
32830007	Wardell	Prevalence and correlates of medicinal cannabis use among adolescents	https://doi.org/10.1016/j.jadohealth.2020.07.032	No
32819963	Dyer	Parents can challenge NICE guidance on medicinal cannabis in court	https://doi.org/10.1136/bmj.m3304	No

(continued)

(continued)

PubMed ID	First author surname	Article title	DOI number	Citation included in the study (yes/no)
32772621	Groh	Medical cannabis and psychiatric disorders: implications for psychiatric nurses	https://doi.org/10.1177/1078390320945791	No
32759172	Narouze	Medical cannabis attitudes and beliefs among pain physicians	https://doi.org/10.1136/rapm-2020-101658	No
32755535	Drosdowsky	Corrigendum to: cancer patients' use of and attitudes towards medicinal cannabis	https://doi.org/10.1071/AH19066_CO	No
32723354	Okusanya	Medical cannabis for the reduction of opioid dosage in the treatment of non-cancer chronic pain: a systematic review	https://doi.org/10.1186/s13643-020-01425-3	No
32717704	Philbin	Medical cannabis laws and medical and non-medical prescription stimulant use among a nationally representative sample of US adults: examining the role of sexual identity and gender	https://doi.org/10.1016/j.drugpo.2020.102861	No
32682602	Takakuwa	Indications and preference considerations for using medical Cannabis in an emergency department: a national survey	https://doi.org/10.1016/j.ajem.2020.07.005	No
32668702	Jerushalmi	Fungal pathogens affecting the production and quality of medical cannabis in israel	https://doi.org/10.3390/plants9070882	No
32662844	Shover	Association of state policies allowing medical cannabis for opioid use disorder with dispensary marketing for this indication	https://doi.org/10.1001/jamanetworkopen.2020.10001	No
32657695	Van Rensburg	Medical cannabis: what practitioners need to know	https://doi.org/10.7196/SAMJ.2020.v110i3.14403	No
32656349	Kaplan	Knowledge, practices, and attitudes of Washington State health care professionals regarding medical cannabis	https://doi.org/10.1089/can.2019.0051	No
32655704	Johal	Medical cannabis for orthopaedic patients with chronic musculoskeletal pain: does evidence support its use?	https://doi.org/10.1177/1759720X20937968	No
32653594	Turna	Overlapping patterns of recreational and medical cannabis use in a large community sample of cannabis users	https://doi.org/10.1016/j.comppsych.2020.152188	No

(continued)

(continued)

PubMed ID	First author surname	Article title	DOI number	Citation included in the study (yes/no)
32640707	Krill	A High-throughput method for the comprehensive analysis of terpenes and terpenoids in medicinal cannabis biomass	https://doi.org/10.3390/metabo10070276	No
32629796	Ramella	Impact of lipid sources on quality traits of medical cannabis-based oil preparations	https://doi.org/10.3390/molecules25132986	No
32600171	Zamengo	Cannabis knowledge and implications for health: considerations regarding the legalization of non-medical cannabis	https://doi.org/10.1177/0025802420934255	No
32581626	Rieder	Authorizing medical cannabis for children	https://doi.org/10.1093/pch/pxaa024	No
32576481	Krediet	Experiences with medical cannabis in the treatment of veterans with PTSD: results from a focus group discussion	https://doi.org/10.1016/j.euroneuro.2020.04.009	Yes
32571806	Wise	Medical cannabis: campaigner calls on home secretary to deliver on access promises	https://doi.org/10.1136/bmj.m2508	No
32570201	Elliott	Barriers in accessing medical cannabis for children with drug-resistant epilepsy in Canada: a qualitative study	https://doi.org/10.1016/j.yebeh.2020.107120	Yes—article was behind a paywall and could not be accessed
32557909	Sznitman	Trends in medical cannabis licensure, Israel, 2013–2018	https://doi.org/10.1111/dar.13116	No
32556203	Safakish	Medical Cannabis for the management of pain and quality of life in chronic pain patients: a prospective observational study	https://doi.org/10.1093/pm/pnaa163	No
32537151	Alexander	Barriers to the wider adoption of medicinal Cannabis	https://doi.org/10.1177/2049463720922884	No
32526965	Aviram	Migraine frequency decrease following prolonged medical cannabis treatment: a cross-sectional study	https://doi.org/10.3390/brainsci10060360	No
32522058	Schlag	Medical cannabis in the UK: from principle to practice	https://doi.org/10.1177/0269881120926677	No
32516686	Zarhin	The trajectory of "medical cannabis" in Israel: driving medicalization in different directions	https://doi.org/10.1016/j.drugpo.2020.102809	No

(continued)

(continued)

PubMed ID	First author surname	Article title	DOI number	Citation included in the study (yes/no)
32513180	Lintzeris	Medical cannabis use in the Australian community following introduction of legal access: the 2018–2019 online cross-sectional cannabis as medicine survey (CAMS-18)	https://doi.org/10.1186/s12954-020-00377-0	No
32507425	Edelstein	Does religiosity matter? University student attitudes and beliefs toward medical cannabis	https://doi.org/10.1016/j.ctim.2020.102407	No
32507423	Gherzi	Safety and pharmacokinetics of medical cannabis preparation in a monocentric series of young patients with drug resistant epilepsy	https://doi.org/10.1016/j.ctim.2020.102402	No
36777304	Benson	Attitudes and knowledge of Australian gastroenterologists around the use of medicinal cannabis for inflammatory bowel disease	https://doi.org/10.1093/crocol/otaa045	No
32499550	Rochfort	Utilisation of design of experiments approach to optimise supercritical fluid extraction of medicinal cannabis	https://doi.org/10.1038/s41598-020-66119-1	No
32429074	Brunetti	Herbal preparations of medical cannabis: a vademecum for prescribing doctors	https://doi.org/10.3390/medicina56050237	No
32404683	Lopez	State medical cannabis laws associated with reduction in opioid prescriptions by orthopaedic surgeons in Medicare Part D Cohort	https://doi.org/10.5435/JAAOS-D-19-00767	No
32404144	Nguyen	Too young for cannabis? Choice of minimum legal age for legalized non-medical cannabis in Canada	https://doi.org/10.1186/s12889-020-08639-z	No
32394570	Humphreys	Recreational cannabis legalization presents an opportunity to reduce the harms of the US medical cannabis industry	https://doi.org/10.1002/wps.20739	No
32394558	Fischer	Considering the health and social welfare impacts of non-medical cannabis legalization	https://doi.org/10.1002/wps.20736	No
32378827	Habib	Sarcoidosis following treatment with medical cannabis		No
32361185	Elliott	Neurologists' perspectives on medical cannabis for pediatric drug-resistant epilepsy in Canada: a qualitative interview study	https://doi.org/10.1016/j.seizure.2020.04.002	No

(continued)

(continued)

PubMed ID	First author surname	Article title	DOI number	Citation included in the study (yes/no)
32353211	Fitzcharles	Medical cannabis use by rheumatology patients following recreational legalization: a prospective observational study of 1000 patients in Canada	https://doi.org/10.1002/acr2.11138	No
32351233	Bougea	Medical cannabis as an alternative therapeutics for Parkinsons' disease: systematic review	https://doi.org/10.1016/j.ctcp.2020.101154	Yes
32349561	Brady	Self-efficacy in researching and obtaining medical cannabis by patients with chronic conditions	https://doi.org/10.1177/1090198120914249	No
34131459	Pawliuk	Efficacy and safety of paediatric medicinal cannabis use: a scoping review	https://doi.org/10.1093/pch/pxaa031	No
32334826	Ryan	Parents' experiences using medical cannabis for their child	https://doi.org/10.1016/j.outlook.2019.12.004	No
32334134	Ternelli	Innovative methods for the preparation of medical cannabis oils with a high content of both cannabinoids and terpenes	https://doi.org/10.1016/j.jpba.2020.113296	No
32325769	Brown	Characteristics of older adults who were early adopters of medical cannabis in the Florida medical Marijuana use registry	https://doi.org/10.3390/jcm9041166	No
32322681	Olla	Evaluation of breath and plasma tetrahydrocannabinol concentration trends postcannabis exposure in medical cannabis patients	https://doi.org/10.1089/can.2018.0070	No
32295931		Correction: cohort study of medical cannabis authorisation and healthcare utilisation in 2014–2017 in Ontario, Canada	https://doi.org/10.1136/jech-2019-212438corr1	No
36777301	Benson	Medicinal Cannabis for inflammatory bowel disease: a survey of perspectives, experiences, and current use in Australian patients	https://doi.org/10.1093/crocol/otaa015	No
32289591	Takakuwa	A history of the society of cannabis clinicians and its contributions and impact on the US medical cannabis movement	https://doi.org/10.1016/j.drugpo.2020.102749	No
32286026	Jarjou'i	Medical cannabis in asthmatic patients		No

(continued)

(continued)

PubMed ID	First author surname	Article title	DOI number	Citation included in the study (yes/no)
32259097	Fischer	Initial indicators of the public health impacts of non-medical cannabis legalization in Canada	https://doi.org/10.1016/j.eclinm.2020.100294	No
32237017	Melnikov	The effect of attitudes, subjective norms and stigma on health-care providers' intention to recommend medicinal cannabis to patients	https://doi.org/10.1111/ijn.12836	No
32227171	Lyon	THC and CBD: is medical cannabis overhyped or under-prescribed?	https://doi.org/10.1093/brain/awaa066	No
32188588	Hurley	Industry's plan to accelerate prescribing of medical cannabis	https://doi.org/10.1136/bmj.m1063	No
32172409	Arboleda	Medical cannabis in supportive cancer care: lessons from Canada	https://doi.org/10.1007/s00520-020-05403-2	No
32163826	Capler	The Medical cannabis standards engagement evaluation and dissemination (SEED) project: a community-based research approach to self-regulating medical cannabis dispensaries in Canada	https://doi.org/10.1016/j.drugpo.2020.102708	No
32116208	Giorgi	Adding medical cannabis to standard analgesic treatment for fibromyalgia: a prospective observational study		No
32114474	Wolfe	Effects of medical and non-medical cannabis use in older adults: protocol for a scoping review	https://doi.org/10.1136/bmjopen-2019-034301	No
32111375	Hergert	Medical cannabis reduced agitation in acquired brain injury: a case study	https://doi.org/10.1016/j.psym.2020.01.006	No
32067838	Takakuwa	The practical knowledge, experience and beliefs of US emergency medicine physicians regarding medical Cannabis: a national survey	https://doi.org/10.1016/j.ajem.2020.01.059	No
32044984	Incze	What should I know about medical cannabis?	https://doi.org/10.1001/jamainternmed.2020.0018	No
32044944	Hill	Medical cannabis	https://doi.org/10.1001/jama.2019.17403	No

(continued)

(continued)

PubMed ID	First author surname	Article title	DOI number	Citation included in the study (yes/no)
32037714	Panozzo	Who is asking about medicinal cannabis in palliative care?	https://doi.org/10.1111/imj.14732	No
32017685	Hergenrather	Cannabinoid and terpenoid doses are associated with adult ADHD status of medical cannabis patients	https://doi.org/10.5041/RMMJ.10384	No
32017680	Aran	Medical cannabis in children	https://doi.org/10.5041/RMMJ.10386	No
32017679	Ben-Zeev	Medical cannabis for intractable epilepsy in childhood: a review	https://doi.org/10.5041/RMMJ.10387	Yes
32016366	Case	The NICE guideline on medicinal cannabis: keeping Pandora's box shut tight?	https://doi.org/10.1093/medlaw/fwaa002	No
32012232	Nugent	Medical cannabis use among individuals with cancer: an unresolved and timely issue	https://doi.org/10.1002/cncr.32732	No
31987225	Gritsenko	Russian Federation medical student knowledge, attitudes and beliefs toward medical cannabis	https://doi.org/10.1016/j.ctim.2019.102274	No
31987223	Benavides	Medical students are unprepared to counsel patients about medical cannabis and want to learn more	https://doi.org/10.1016/j.ctim.2019.102237	No
31984702	Appiani	Medical cannabis: risks related to its indication prior to approval	https://doi.org/10.5546/aap.2020.eng.64	No
31977646	Shimol	Development of Raynaud phenomenon following use of medical cannabis	https://doi.org/10.1097/RHU.0000000000001312	No
31977375	Mohiuddin	Adherence to consolidated standards of reporting trials (CONSORT) guidelines for reporting safety outcomes in trials of medical cannabis and cannabis-based medicines for chronic noncancer pain: a systematic review	https://doi.org/10.1097/AJP.0000000000000807	No
31959585	Sznitman	Medical cannabis and insomnia in older adults with chronic pain: a cross-sectional study	https://doi.org/10.1136/bmjspcare-2019-001938	No
31959279	Drosdowsky	Cancer patients' use of and attitudes towards medicinal cannabis	https://doi.org/10.1071/AH19066	No

(continued)

(continued)

PubMed ID	First author surname	Article title	DOI number	Citation included in the study (yes/no)
31948424	Sarris	Medicinal cannabis for psychiatric disorders: a clinically-focused systematic review	https://doi.org/10.1186/s12888-019-2409-8	Yes
31945040	Oldfield	Medical cannabis: knowledge and expectations in a cohort of North Island New Zealand general practitioners		Yes—article was behind a paywall and could not be accessed
34676342	Schlag	An evaluation of regulatory regimes of medical cannabis: what lessons can be learned for the UK?	https://doi.org/10.1159/000505028	No
31895183	Téllez-Zenteno	Medical cannabis as a treatment for patients with epilepsy, sleep disorders, and posttraumatic stress disorder	https://doi.org/10.1097/WNP.0000000000000650	Yes—article was behind a paywall and could not be accessed
31892011	Pichini	Fast and sensitive UHPLC-MS/MS analysis of cannabinoids and their acid precursors in pharmaceutical preparations of medical cannabis and their metabolites in conventional and non-conventional biological matrices of treated individual	https://doi.org/10.1016/j.talanta.2019.120537	No
31891265	Linciano	Isolation of a high-affinity cannabinoid for the human CB1 receptor from a medicinal *Cannabis sativa* variety: Δ(9)-tetrahydrocannabutol, the butyl homologue of Δ(9)-tetrahydrocannabinol	https://doi.org/10.1021/acs.jnatprod.9b00876	No
31887404	Karim	Medical cannabis authorization in patients with cancer in the prelegalization era: a population-based study	https://doi.org/10.1016/j.jpainsymman.2019.12.367	No
31864106	Fischer	Emerging prospects for non-medical cannabis legalisation in New Zealand: an initial view and contextualization	https://doi.org/10.1016/j.drugpo.2019.102632	No
31852743	Glickman	Prescribing medical cannabis: ethical considerations for primary care providers	https://doi.org/10.1136/medethics-2019-105759	No
31831619	Eurich	Cohort study of medical cannabis authorisation and healthcare utilisation in 2014–2017 in Ontario, Canada	https://doi.org/10.1136/jech-2019-212438	No

(continued)

(continued)

PubMed ID	First author surname	Article title	DOI number	Citation included in the study (yes/no)
31831352	Gladden	Arkansas community's attitudes toward the regulation of medical cannabis and the pharmacist's involvement in Arkansas medical cannabis	https://doi.org/10.1016/j.japh.2019.11.005	No
31800438	Kleeman-Forsthuber	Medicinal Cannabis in orthopaedic practice	https://doi.org/10.5435/JAAOS-D-19-00438	No
31790276	Olla	Short-term effects of cannabis consumption on cognitive performance in medical cannabis patients	https://doi.org/10.1080/23279095.2019.1681424	No
31747851	Wadsworth	Mental health and medical cannabis use among youth and young adults in Canada	https://doi.org/10.1080/10826084.2019.1691594	No
31743746	Portman	Medical cannabis as an effective treatment for refractory symptoms of paraneoplastic stiff person syndrome	https://doi.org/10.1016/j.jpainsymman.2019.11.007	No
31740295	Philbrick	Up in smoke: one state's perspective on the affordability of medical cannabis	https://doi.org/10.1016/j.japh.2019.09.008	No
31731110	de Carvalho Reis	Efficacy and adverse event profile of cannabidiol and medicinal cannabis for treatment-resistant epilepsy: systematic review and meta-analysis	https://doi.org/10.1016/j.yebeh.2019.106635	Yes—article was behind a paywall and could not be accessed
31706799	Cáceres Guido	Medicinal cannabis in Latin America: history, current state of regulation, and the role of the pharmacist in a new clinical experience with cannabidiol oil	https://doi.org/10.1016/j.japh.2019.09.012	No
31693457	Bruce	Perceived efficacy of medical cannabis in the treatment of co-occurring health-related quality of life symptoms	https://doi.org/10.1080/08964289.2019.1683712	No
31658906	Strawhacker	Medical cannabis and school: separating fact from fiction	https://doi.org/10.1177/1942602X19877561	No
31600630	Lancione	Non-medical cannabis in North America: an overview of regulatory approaches	https://doi.org/10.1016/j.puhe.2019.08.018	No
31585701	Moeller	A nationwide survey of pharmacy students' knowledge and perceptions regarding medical cannabis	https://doi.org/10.1016/j.japh.2019.08.008	No

(continued)

(continued)

PubMed ID	First author surname	Article title	DOI number	Citation included in the study (yes/no)
31560957	Boehnke	High-frequency medical cannabis use is associated with worse pain among individuals with chronic pain	https://doi.org/10.1016/j.jpain.2019.09.006	No
31539298	Zarrabi	Perception of benefits and harms of medical cannabis among seriously ill patients in an outpatient palliative care practice	https://doi.org/10.1089/jpm.2019.0211	No
31535218	Maharajan	Medical cannabis for chronic pain: can it make a difference in pain management?	https://doi.org/10.1007/s00540-019-02680-y	No
31479044	Dryburgh	Using therapeutic drug monitoring and pharmacovigilance to overcome some of the challenges of developing medicinal cannabis from botanical origins	https://doi.org/10.1097/FTD.0000000000000698	No
31389860	Pichini	Δ9-tetrahydrocannabinol and cannabidiol time courses in the sera of "light cannabis" smokers: discriminating light cannabis use from illegal and medical cannabis use	https://doi.org/10.1097/FTD.0000000000000683	No
31190678	Sznitman	Long-term medical cannabis use and risk factors for diversion: report on physician's guidance and patients' behaviour	https://doi.org/10.1017/S1478951519000348	No

Notes

- PubMed search conducted on 30 December 2023
- Search terms were (*"medicinal cannabis"* [Title]) OR (*"medical cannabis"* [Title])
- Date range of citations retrieved: 1 January 2020 to 31 December 2023
- Language of citations: English
- Number of records retrieved: 683 records

Appendix C
Studies Reviewed by Sarris et al. (2020)

Mental disorder[a]	Cannabinoid(s) studied	Methodology	Results	Clinical comment
Social anxiety				
Bergamaschi et al. (2011)	CBD (600 mg)	24 treatment-naïve patients with social anxiety were blindly allocated to receive CBD or placebo 1.5 h before a simulated public speaking test. 12 unmedicated healthy controls also completed the test. Self-reports on the visual analogue mood scale, and negative self-statement scale, and physiological measures were taken at six time points during the test	Pre-test CBD administration in social anxiety patients versus placebo, resulted in significantly reduced anxiety, cognitive impairment and discomfort in speech performance, and significantly decreased hyper-alertness in anticipatory speech. CBD and control groups however did not differ, reflecting similar response profiles during the public speaking test	The initial positive studies suggest that CBD may be a beneficial safe option (a larger confirmatory study needed)
Crippa et al. (2011)	CBD (400 mg)	Compared regional cerebral blood flow activity in 10 treatment-naïve patients with SAD who were given CBD or placebo, in a double-blinded crossover manner	CBD compared to placebo, resulted in significantly lower subjective anxiety, and modulated blood flow in the left parahippocampal gyrus, hippocampus, and inferior temporal gyrus, and right posterior cingulate gyrus	

(continued)

G. Bennett, *A Scoping Review of Clinical Studies About the Therapeutic Benefits of Medical Cannabis*, https://doi.org/10.1007/978-981-97-7941-3

(continued)

Mental disorder[a]	Cannabinoid(s) studied	Methodology	Results	Clinical comment
Post-traumatic stress disorder (PTSD)				
Greer et al. (2014)	Cannabis (not defined)	Analysed retrospectively collected CAPS data from 80 patients with PTSD	Patients reported > 75% decrease in CAPS scores when they were using cannabis compared to periods when they were not	No firm evidence yet, however initial case analyses suggest this application may be of benefit to manage PTSD symptoms, reduce anxiety, and improve sleep
Elms et al. (2019)	CBD (capsule or spray; mean dosage at week-8 of 49 mg)	Open label retrospective case study data from 11 adult patients with PTSD. Data assessed over 8 weeks	Mean PTSD symptoms on the PCL-5 reduced by 28%. Actual statistical data analysis not conducted	
Depression				
Portenoy et al. (2012)	Nabiximols: THC (2.7 mg) and CBD (2.5 mg)	263 patients with advanced cancer and opioid-refractory pain were randomly allocated to receive placebo or nabiximols daily at low (1–4 sprays), medium (6–10 sprays) or high (11–16 sprays) doses, for 5 weeks. Pre/ post-measures included average pain, worst pain, sleep disruption, quality of life and mood	Reports of pain relief were significantly greater for nabiximols than placebo overall, especially in the low- and medium-dose groups. There were no other significant group differences. Adverse events were dose-related with only the high-dose group reporting a decrease in mood	No evidence for use in depression, however higher doses of THC-predominant medicines may in fact lower mood
Insomnia				
Shannon and Opila-Lehman (2016)	CBD capsules (25 mg) + liquid (6–25 mg)	Patient (10 y.o. girl with prior early childhood trauma) was prescribed fish oil (750 mg daily) + 1 CBD oil capsule daily for 5 months. CBD liquid (12–24 mg) was added to the regime for 1 month and reduced to 6–12 mg p.r.n (or 'when needed'). Sleep assessed monthly via SDSC	SDSC scores decreased over the 5-month period, indicating an increase in sleep quality and quantity	Only case study and secondary outcome evidence at present. Encouraging as a potential use pending controlled studies, however next-day effects need to be assessed in terms of somnolence and cognitive functioning
Johnson et al. (2013)	Nabiximols: THC (2.7 mg) and CBD (2.5 mg) OR THC only (2.7 mg)	43 patients, with advanced cancer and opioid-refractory pain, self-administered daily nabiximols or THC-only sprays for 5 weeks. Safety, tolerability, pain and quality of life were assessed	Across groups, pain decreased at every visit, and showed pre-/post improvement with insomnia and fatigue	

(continued)

(continued)

Mental disorder[a]	Cannabinoid(s) studied	Methodology	Results	Clinical comment
Shannon et al. (2019)	CBD capsules (mainly 25 mg/ day)	A retrospective case series of 72 adults given CBD for anxiety and sleep complaints at a psychiatric clinic, as an adjunct to usual treatment. Assessed monthly over 12 weeks	Anxiety scores on the HAMA decreased within the first month in 79% of the sample and remained decreased during the study duration. PSQI sleep score improved within the first month in 67%, but fluctuated over time. Data appeared to not be statistically significant for the group presenting with a primary complaint of anxiety (those with sleep disturbance fared better)	
Schizophrenia				
Leweke et al. (2012)	CBD (600–800 mg)	42 individuals with schizophrenia were randomly assigned to receive 600–800 mg of CBD or amisulpride over 4 weeks. The PANSS and BPRS were administered every 14 days. Blood was also collected	Both treatments were effective in reducing PANSS and BPRS scores at each time point. CBD was tolerated better, with fewer side effects reported. Anandamide levels were higher in the CBD group post-treatment	Avoid any use of high THC in youth. 600 mg–1200 mg of CBD per day may be effective as an adjunct for +ve and −ve symptoms
McGuire et al. (2018)	CBD (1000 mg)	88 antipsychotic-treated patients with schizophrenia were randomly given placebo or CBD alongside existing medication for 6 weeks. Pre/post-trial measures included the PANSS, brief assessment of cognition in schizophrenia, global assessment of functioning, clinical global impressions of improvement and severity scales	The CBD group reported lower positive symptom scores, and were more likely to be rated as improved and less severely ill than the placebo group. The CBD group also showed improvements in the cognitive domain of motor speed compared to placebo. CBD was tolerated well with similar adverse event rates reported between the groups	
Boggs et al. (2018)	CBD (600 mg)	36 individuals with schizophrenia were randomised to receive CBD or placebo adjunctively to current antipsychotic medication for 6 weeks. PANSS and MCCB were assessed pre/ post-trial	Both groups showed improvement on PANSS scores and only the placebo group improved on the MCCB. Similar side effects were noted between the groups, with more sedation evident in the CBD group	

(continued)

(continued)

Mental disorder[a]	Cannabinoid(s) studied	Methodology	Results	Clinical comment
Bipolar disorder				
Zuardi et al. (2010)	CBD (600–1200 mg)	Two patients with bipolar I disorder were administered CBD for 30 days with 5 days of placebo pre/post-trial. Patients were assessed on the YMRS and BPRS every 7 days	One patient showed improvements in YMRS and BPRS scores while on CBD plus olanzapine but no additional improvement during CBD monotherapy. The second patient had no symptom improvement with any dose of CBD. Both tolerated CBD well with no side effects reported	Not presently recommended. CBD appears not to be effective in attenuating mania
Attention deficit hyperactivity disorder (ADHD)				
Cooper et al. (2017)	Nabiximols: THC (2.7 mg) and CBD (2.5 mg)	30 adults with ADHD were randomly prescribed nabiximols or placebo for 6 weeks. A participant's optimal dose was decided at day 14. The QBT assessed cognitive performance and activity level (head movements), conners adult ADHD rating scale rated ADHD symptoms, and self-reports to examine emotional lability	The nabiximols group showed an improvement in QBT scores that approached significance. Nominally significant improvements in ADHD symptoms were also found for the nabiximols group compared to placebo	Potentially may be effective in managing some ADHD symptoms however more research is needed. Lower THC formulas alleviate concerns about cognitive impairment

Notes [a]First Author; *THC* tetrahydrocannabinol, *CBD* cannabidiol, *QBT* quantitative behavioural test, *PANSS* positive and negative syndrome scale, *MCCB* MATRICS consensus cognitive battery, *HAMA* Hamilton anxiety rating scale, *PSQI* Pittsburgh sleep quality index, *YMRS* young mania rating scale, *BPRS* brief psychiatric rating scale, *SDSC* sleep disturbance scale for children, *CAPS* clinician administered posttraumatic scale; PLC-5 = PTSD checklist for DSM-5
Source Sarris et al. (2020, pp. 4–5)

References

Bergamaschi, M. M., Queiroz, R. H., Chagas, M. H., de Oliveira, D. C., De Martinis, B. S., Kapczinski, F., Quevedo, J., Roesler, R., Schröder, N., Nardi, A. E., Martín-Santos, R., Hallak, J. E., Zuardi, A. W., & Crippa, J. A. (2011). Cannabidiol reduces the anxiety induced by simulated public speaking in treatment-naïve social phobia patients. *Neuropsychopharmacology: Official Publication of the American College of Neuropsychopharmacology, 36*(6), 1219–1226. https://doi.org/10.1038/npp.2011.6

Boggs, D. L., Surti, T., Gupta, A., Gupta, S., Niciu, M., Pittman, B., Schnakenberg Martin, A. M., Thurnauer, H., Davies, A., D'Souza, D. C., & Ranganathan, M. (2018). The effects of cannabidiol (CBD) on cognition and symptoms in outpatients with chronic schizophrenia a randomized placebo controlled trial. *Psychopharmacology, 235*(7), 1923–1932. https://doi.org/10.1007/s00213-018-4885-9

Cooper, R. E., Williams, E., Seegobin, S., Tye, C., Kuntsi, J., & Asherson, P. (2017). Cannabinoids in attention-deficit/hyperactivity disorder: A randomised-controlled trial. *European neuropsychopharmacology: The Journal of the European College of Neuropsychopharmacology, 27*(8), 795–808. https://doi.org/10.1016/j.euroneuro.2017.05.005

Crippa, J. A. S., Derenusson, G. N., Ferrari, T. B., Wichert-Ana, L., Duran, F. L., Martin-Santos, R., … & Hallak, J. E. C. (2011). Neural basis of anxiolytic effects of cannabidiol (CBD) in generalized social anxiety disorder: a preliminary report. *Journal of Psychopharmacology, 25*(1), 121–130. https://doi.org/10.1177/0269881110379283

Elms, L., Shannon, S., Hughes, S., & Lewis, N. (2019). Cannabidiol in the treatment of post-traumatic stress disorder: A case series. *Journal of Alternative and Complementary Medicine (New York, N.Y.), 25*(4), 392–397. https://doi.org/10.1089/acm.2018.0437

Greer, G. R., Grob, C. S., & Halberstadt, A. L. (2014). PTSD symptom reports of patients evaluated for the New Mexico Medical Cannabis Program. *Journal of Psychoactive Drugs, 46*(1), 73–77. https://doi.org/10.1080/02791072.2013.873843

Johnson, J. R., Lossignol, D., Burnell-Nugent, M., & Fallon, M. T. (2013). An open-label extension study to investigate the long-term safety and tolerability of THC/CBD oromucosal spray and oromucosal THC spray in patients with terminal cancer-related pain refractory to strong opioid analgesics. *Journal of Pain and Symptom Management, 46*(2), 207–218. https://doi.org/10.1016/j.jpainsymman.2012.07.014

Leweke, F. M., Piomelli, D., Pahlisch, F., Muhl, D., Gerth, C. W., Hoyer, C., Klosterkötter, J., Hellmich, M., & Koethe, D. (2012). Cannabidiol enhances anandamide signaling and alleviates psychotic symptoms of schizophrenia. *Translational Psychiatry, 2*(3), e94. https://doi.org/10.1038/tp.2012.15

McGuire, P., Robson, P., Cubala, W. J., Vasile, D., Morrison, P. D., Barron, R., Taylor, A., & Wright, S. (2018). Cannabidiol (CBD) as an adjunctive therapy in Schizophrenia: A multicenter randomized controlled trial. *The American Journal of Psychiatry, 175*(3), 225–231. https://doi.org/10.1176/appi.ajp.2017.17030325

Portenoy, R. K., Ganae-Motan, E. D., Allende, S., Yanagihara, R., Shaiova, L., Weinstein, S., McQuade, R., Wright, S., & Fallon, M. T. (2012). Nabiximols for opioid-treated cancer patients with poorly-controlled chronic pain: A randomized, placebo-controlled, graded-dose trial. *The Journal of Pain, 13*(5), 438–449. https://doi.org/10.1016/j.jpain.2012.01.003

Sarris, J., Sinclair, J., Karamacoska, D., Davidson, M., & Firth, J. (2020). Medicinal cannabis for psychiatric disorders: a clinically-focused systematic review. *BMC Psychiatry, 20*(1), 24. https://doi.org/10.1186/s12888-019-2409-8

Shannon, S., & Opila-Lehman, J. (2016). Effectiveness of cannabidiol oil for pediatric anxiety and insomnia as part of posttraumatic stress disorder: A case report. *The Permanente Journal, 20*(4), 16-005. https://doi.org/10.7812/TPP/16-005

Shannon, S., Lewis, N., Lee, H., & Hughes, S. (2019). Cannabidiol in Anxiety and sleep: A large case series. *The Permanente Journal, 23*, 18-041. https://doi.org/10.7812/TPP/18-041

Zuardi, A., Crippa, J., Dursun, S., Morais, S., Vilela, J., Sanches, R., & Hallak, J. (2010). Cannabidiol was ineffective for manic episode of bipolar affective disorder. *Journal of Psychopharmacology (Oxford, England), 24*(1), 135–137. https://doi.org/10.1177/0269881108096521

Appendix D
A Summary of the Studies Evaluating the Efficacy of Medicinal Cannabis Preparations for Mental Health and Neurodevelopmental Conditions

Study	CBD preparation	Study design	Study population	Findings
Bar-Lev Schleider et al. (2019)	Most patients: Cannabis oil with a THC:CBD ratio of 1:20 (30% CBD, 1.5% THC) Participants with a history of sensitivity to prior medications: Cannabis oil with a THC: CBD ratio of 1:20 (15% CBD, 0.75% THC) Participants with severe sleep disturbance or significant aggressive behaviour: addition of 3% THC oil following initial treatment phase	Prospective cohort study (outcome measurement at 6 months)	Autistic children and adolescents ($n = 188$)	Following 6 months of treatment, 60% of participants were assessed ($n = 93$), of which 28 patients (30.1%) reported a significant improvement, 50 (53.7%) moderate, 6 (6.4%) slight and 8 (8.6%) had no change in their condition' (Bar-Lev Schleider et al., 2019). Additionally, 28 patients (30%) reported adverse effects, including restlessness
Cooper et al. (2017)	Sativex oromucosal spray (1:1 ratio; delta-9-tetrahydrocannabinol to cannabidiol)	Double-blind randomised placebo-controlled trial (outcome measurement at day 42)	Adults with ADHD ($n = 30$)	No significant difference from placebo with respect to cognitive performance and activity level, inattention or emotional lability. Nominally significant improvements in hyperactivity/ impulsivity ($p = 0.03$) and inhibition ($p = 0.05$), though these findings did not reach the threshold for significance after adjustment for multiple testing
Rifkin-Zybutz et al. (2023)	Variable cannabis-based medical products	Cohort study (outcome measurement at 1, 3 and 6 months)	Patients with generalised anxiety disorders ($n = 302$)	Significant improvements in anxiety, sleep quality and quality of life at all three time points were reported ($p < 0.001$)

(continued)

G. Bennett, *A Scoping Review of Clinical Studies About the Therapeutic Benefits of Medical Cannabis*, https://doi.org/10.1007/978-981-97-7941-3

(continued)

Study	CBD preparation	Study design	Study population	Findings
Sarris et al. (2020)	Variable preparations used in constituent studies	Systematic review	Patients with major psychiatric disorders (13 eligible studies)	Depression: No benefit from delta-9-tetrahydrocannabinol Mania: no benefit from CBD PTSD: weak evidence from case studies Schizophrenia: mixed evidence for use as an adjunctive treatment Social anxiety: tentative support for CBD Sleep disorders: weak evidence from case studies
Silva Junior et al. (2022)	Variable preparations used in constituent studies	Systematic review	Autistic patients (nine eligible studies)	Some eligible studies reported reductions in the frequency and/ or intensity of various symptoms, 'including hyperactivity, attacks of self-mutilation and anger, sleep problems, anxiety, restlessness, psychomotor agitation, irritability, aggressiveness, perseverance and depression', as well as improvements in 'cognition, sensory sensitivity, attention, social interaction, and language' (Silva Junior et al., 2021) Adverse effects included 'sleep disorders, restlessness, nervousness and change in appetite' (Silva Junior et al., 2021)
Timler et al. (2023)	'A mix of THC and CBD (3:2 ratio; 25 mg/ml THC; 17 mg/ml CBD)'. (Timler et al., 2023)	Double-blind randomised placebo-controlled crossover trial (outcome measurement at 18 weeks)	Adults diagnosed with dementia based in residential care facilities (*n* = 21)	No significant difference from placebo with respect to behaviour, quality of life and pain. However, a significant difference was found with respect to agitation, in favour of the treatment group

Source Korb et al. (2023, p. 1204)

References

Bar-Lev Schleider, L., Mechoulam, R., Saban, N., Meiri, G., & Novack, V. (2019). Real life experience of medical cannabis treatment in autism: Analysis of safety and efficacy. *Scientific Reports*, *9*(1), 200. https://doi.org/10.1038/s41598-018-37570-y

Cooper, R. E., Williams, E., Seegobin, S., Tye, C., Kuntsi, J., & Asherson, P. (2017). Cannabinoids in attention-deficit/hyperactivity disorder: A randomised-controlled trial. *European Neuropsychopharmacology: The Journal of the European College of Neuropsychopharmacology, 27*(8), 795–808. https://doi.org/10.1016/j.euroneuro.2017.05.005

Korb, L., Tromans, S., Perera, B., Khan, N., Burrows, L., Laugharne, R., Hassiotis, A., Allgar, V., Efron, D., Maidment, I., & Shankar, R. (2023). The potential for medicinal cannabis to help manage challenging behaviour in people with intellectual disability: A perspective review. *Journal of psychopharmacology (Oxford, England), 37*(12), 1201–1208. https://doi.org/10.1177/02698811231209192

Rifkin-Zybutz, R., Erridge, S., Holvey, C., Coomber, R., Gaffney, J., Lawn, W., Barros, D., Bhoskar, U., Mwimba, G., Praveen, K., Symeon, C., Sachdeva-Mohan, S., Rucker, J. J., & Sodergren, M. H. (2023). Clinical outcome data of anxiety patients treated with cannabis-based medicinal products in the United Kingdom: a cohort study from the UK Medical Cannabis Registry. *Psychopharmacology, 240*(8), 1735–1745. https://doi.org/10.1007/s00213-023-06399-3

Sarris, J., Sinclair, J., Karamacoska, D., Davidson, M., & Firth, J. (2020). Medicinal cannabis for psychiatric disorders: a clinically-focused systematic review. *BMC Psychiatry, 20*(1), 24. https://doi.org/10.1186/s12888-019-2409-8

Silva, E. A. D., Junior, Medeiros, W. M. B., Torro, N., Sousa, J. M. M., Almeida, I. B. C. M., Costa, F. B. D., Pontes, K. M., Nunes, E. L. G., Rosa, M. D. D., & Albuquerque, K. L. G. D. (2022). Cannabis and cannabinoid use in autism spectrum disorder: A systematic review. *Trends in Psychiatry and Psychotherapy, 44*, e20200149. https://doi.org/10.47626/2237-6089-2020-0149

Timler, A., Bulsara, C., Bulsara, M., Vickery, A., Jacques, A., & Codde, J. (2023). Examining the use of cannabidiol and delta-9-tetrahydrocannabinol-based medicine among individuals diagnosed with dementia living within residential aged care facilities: Results of a double-blind randomised crossover trial. *Australasian Journal on Ageing, 42*(4), 698–709. https://doi.org/10.1111/ajag.13224

Appendix E
Studies Reviewed by Rønne et al. (2021)

G. Bennett, *A Scoping Review of Clinical Studies About the Therapeutic Benefits of Medical Cannabis*, https://doi.org/10.1007/978-981-97-7941-3

Reference	Country	Objective	Study population and methods	Results/conclusion	Comments
Philpot et al. (2019)	USA (Minnesota)	To explore the attitudes, beliefs, and knowledge of healthcare providers in order to identify ongoing barriers, biases and knowledge gaps relating to medical cannabis	62 providers answered a questionnaire (response rate: 31%). 76% of respondents were physicians	Experiences: 27.4% was registered to certify patients for medical cannabis, but one half reported having patients who had been certified for medical cannabis. 10% of providers had been certifying patients, and the mean number of patients certified was 4 Attitudes and beliefs: 58.1% of the providers believed that medical cannabis was a legitimate medical therapy, and 38.7% believed that providers should be offering it to patients for managing medical conditions. 50% of providers were not ready to or did not want to answer patient questions about medical cannabis, and 77.4% of providers were interested in learning more about it. A majority (> 50%) of providers believed that medical cannabis was helpful for treating the qualifying medical conditions of cancer, terminal illness, and intractable pain. A majority of providers did not know if medical cannabis was effective for managing nearly one-half of the other state designated qualifying medical conditions. Few believed that medical cannabis improved quality of life domains. 38,7% of providers believed that medical cannabis interacted with medical therapies	Minnesota has created a medical cannabis comprehensive program, and enrolled patients has access to extracted cannabis products in liquid or oil form

(continued)

(continued)

Reference	Country	Objective	Study population and methods	Results/conclusion	Comments
Braun et al. (2018)	USA	To explore medical oncologists' attitudes and knowledge in relation to prescription of medical cannabis and to explore its comparative effectiveness and risks	237 medical oncologists answered a questionnaire (response rate: 63%) The study explored whether oncologists reported discussing medical marijuana with patients, recommended it clinically and felt sufficiently informed to make such recommendations. The study also explored medical marijuana's comparative effectiveness for several conditions and its risks compared with prescription of opioids	Experiences: 80% conducted discussions about MM with patients or their families, and 46% recommended MM clinically Attitudes and beliefs: 30% of oncologists felt sufficiently informed to make recommendations regarding MM. More than half of oncologists who reported recommending MM did not consider themselves to have sufficient knowledge to make a recommendation. 67% viewed it as a helpful adjunct to standard pain management strategies, and 65% thought MM is equally or more effective than standard treatments for anorexia and cachexia	It was legal for physicians to prescribe medical cannabis in 30 states and the District of Columbia

(continued)

(continued)

Reference	Country	Objective	Study population and methods	Results/conclusion	Comments
Luba et al. (2018)	USA (46 states)	To examine palliative and hospice care providers' attitudes and beliefs regarding the use of cannabis for terminally ill populations	426 palliative and hospice care providers, (345 medical doctors, 58 nurses, and 23 others) answered a questionnaire (response rate was not reported)	Attitudes and beliefs: 70% of all participants reported that cannabis could aid in end-of-life care. When examining individual symptoms, almost 90% believed that cannabis could be helpful in treating nausea, appetite loss and pain, almost 70% believed it could be helpful in the treatment of sleep problems, almost 60% in the treatment of irritability and emotional suffering. More than half of the study participants believed that adverse effects of cannabis would be equally or less problematic than conventional treatments when considering pain, appetite loss, nausea, sleep, and end-of-life care. 61% of all participants would recommend cannabis to patients with a terminal illness. More than half would recommend it for the treatment of appetite loss, nausea and pain	Respondents were from 46 different states. 45.3% of respondents were from states where cannabis was illegal, 36.2% were from states where cannabis was legal for medical use, and 22.1% were from states where cannabis was legal for recreational use. No further details on the prescription procedure or law on medical cannabis in each state were described

(continued)

(continued)

Reference	Country	Objective	Study population and methods	Results/conclusion	Comments
Robinson et al. (2018)	USA	To explore the extent of dermatologists' familiarity with and interest in cannabinoids as therapeutics	531 dermatologists answered a questionnaire (response rate: 21.3%)	Experiences: 55% reported at least one patient-initiated discussion about cannabinoids in the last year Attitudes and beliefs: 86% thought cannabinoids should be legal for medical treatment. Around 94% believed research into dermatologic uses of cannabinoids is worthwhile. 86% were willing to prescribe an approved cannabinoid as a topical treatment, and 71% were willing to prescribe an oral form. 64% did not know that cannabidiol is not psychoactive, and 29% did not know that tetrahydrocannabinol is psychoactive	See the chapter "Procedures and definitions of medical cannabis prescriptions in included studies"

(continued)

(continued)

Reference	Country	Objective	Study population and methods	Results/conclusion	Comments
Sideris et al. (2018)	USA (New York)	To probe physicians' knowledge and perspectives of the New York State Medical Marijuana Programme (NY-MMP) and cannabinoids in patient care	164 physicians with various specialties answered a questionnaire (response rate was not reported). 13% of the physicians were registered with the MMP, which authorized them to recommend medial cannabis	Experiences: 95% of registered physicians and 49% of nonregistered physicians had patients who inquired about medical cannabis within the past year. More than 75% reported having patients who used cannabis for symptom control. 25% of all respondents had recommended synthetic cannabinoid drugs, which were approved by the Food and Drug Administration, for patients Attitudes and beliefs: 71% believed that medical cannabis should be an option available to patients. 55% reported a willingness to discuss medical cannabis with patients if they felt their patients could benefit	Medical cannabis was legal in the state of New York; physicians can certify that patients have a qualifying condition and may recommend medical cannabis but cannot issue a prescription. To recommend medical cannabis, physicians must be registered with the NY-MMP, including a 4-h course which provides an overview of adverse effects, guidelines for dosing and administration etc.

(continued)

(continued)

Reference	Country	Objective	Study population and methods	Results/conclusion	Comments
Bega et al. (2017)	USA (14 states)	To gather data on cannabis-related prescribing practices and views regarding potential risks and benefits of medical cannabis among neurologists caring for patients with Parkinson's disease	56 neurologists answered a questionnaire (response rate: 63%)	Experiences: 80% of all respondents reported having patients using medical cannabis (not described if they used it legally or illegally), and 95% had been requested to prescribe it. 10% of all respondents had recommended the use of cannabis to their patients. 23% reported having formal education on medical cannabis (not defined) Attitudes and beliefs: 93% expected medical cannabis to be effective for appetite loss, 85% for pain, 80% for nausea, and 67% for anxiety. More than half expected that medical cannabis would worsen motivation, sleepiness, balance, forgetfulness, and hallucinations	Medical cannabis was legal in eight of the surveyed states and illegal in six of the states. No further details of the law on medical cannabis were described

(continued)

(continued)

Reference	Country	Objective	Study population and methods	Results/conclusion	Comments
Mathern et al. (2015)	USA (study population was primarily from North America and Europe)	To study opinions about the use of medical cannabis for people with epilepsy among physicians, other health professionals and patients/the public. (Only results from physicians are included in this review)	609 (140 epileptologists, 31 general neurologists, 9 general physicians, 36 basic researchers, 40 nurses and 353 patients/public) from different countries answered a questionnaire (response rate not reported as participants were not invited individually). Only results on health professionals are presented in this review The study compared epileptologists/ neurologists and other physicians	Attitudes and beliefs: fewer epileptologists/ neurologists supported the use of medical cannabis in the treatment of people with epilepsy compared with general medical personal	Law on medical cannabis was not described. See the chapter "procedures and definitions of medical cannabis prescriptions in included studies"

(continued)

(continued)

Reference	Country	Objective	Study population and methods	Results/conclusion	Comments
Kondrad and Reid (2013)	USA (Colorado)	To study physicians' attitudes towards medical cannabis	520 general practitioners (GPs) answered a questionnaire (response rate of 30%) The study compared physicians with and without experiences of prescribing medical cannabis to patients	Experiences: 31% had ever recommended medical cannabis, primary to treat pain, muscle spasms and nausea. GPs reported a need for continuing medical education about medical cannabis Attitudes and beliefs: those who had recommended medical cannabis were significantly more likely to be convinced of its benefits and less concerned about its risks than physicians who had never recommended it (72% vs. 26% respectively ($p < 0.001$))	In Colorado, physicians could certify a patient registry card allowing patients to use cannabis for medical conditions
Charuvastra et al. (2005)	USA	To investigate physicians' practices and attitudes regarding the use of medical cannabis	960 physicians (various specialities; addiction medicine/ psychiatry, family practice, general psychiatry, internal medicine, obstetrics and gynaecology) answered a questionnaire (response rate: 66%) The study compared physicians specialized in addiction medicine with other specialties	Attitudes and beliefs: 36% reported that physicians should be able to prescribe medical cannabis legally. Compared to physicians specialized in addiction medicine (referent), internists and obstetrician/gynaecologists were significantly more likely to support medical use of cannabis, OR: 1.62 (1.01–2.50) and OR: 2.21 (1.39–3.53 respectively)	Law on medical cannabis was not described. See the chapter "procedures and definitions of medical cannabis prescriptions in included studies"

(continued)

(continued)

Reference	Country	Objective	Study population and methods	Results/conclusion	Comments
Jacobs et al. (2019)	Australia	To assess Australian psychiatrists' and psychiatry trainees' knowledge about and attitudes towards medicinal cannabinoids, given the recent relaxation of cannabinoid-prescribing laws in Australia	88 physicians responded to an online accessible survey, with 55 completing all items, 23 psychiatrists and 32 trainees (response rate: 1.1%)	Attitudes and beliefs: 54% of respondents would prescribe medical cannabinoids if it was legal for them to do so (trainees did not have the authority). Participants believed there was evidence for the use of cannabidiol and tetrahydrocannabinol in treating childhood epilepsy, chronic pain, and nausea and vomiting. Generally, they were poor at differentiating between indications for cannabidiol versus tetrahydrocannabinol. They were most concerned about medicinal cannabinoids leading to psychotic symptoms, addiction and dependence, apathy and recreational use	In Australia there was legal access to medical cannabis for patients approved for it by a physician

(continued)

(continued)

Reference	Country	Objective	Study population and methods	Results/conclusion	Comments
Karanges et al. (2018)	Australia	To examine the knowledge and attitudes of Australian GPs towards medical cannabis, including patient demands, GP perceptions of therapeutic effects and potential harms, perceived knowledge and willingness to prescribe	640 GPs answered a questionnaire (response rate 37%) Distribution of printed questionnaires at one-day general practice educational seminars held in five major Australian Cities	Experience: (61.5%) reported one or more patient enquiries about medical cannabis in the last 3 months Attitudes and beliefs: Most felt that their own knowledge was inadequate and only 28.8% felt comfortable discussing medical cannabis with patients. Over half (56.5%) supported availability on prescription, with the preferred access model involving trained GPs prescribing independently of specialists. Support for use of medical cannabis was condition-specific, with strong support for use in cancer pain, palliative care and epilepsy, and much lower support for use in depression and anxiety	In Australia there was legal access to medical cannabis for patients approved for it by a physician
Irvine (2006)	Australia	To examine GPs' attitudes to and knowledge of medical cannabis	32 GPs answered a questionnaire (response rate not reported)	Attitudes and beliefs: 75% of the sample would be prepared to prescribe medical cannabis if it was legal, supported by peers and based on good-quality clinical research evidence	In Australia, medical cannabis was illegal at the time

(continued)

(continued)

Reference	Country	Objective	Study population and methods	Results/conclusion	Comments
St-Amant et al. (2015)	Canada (Quebec)	To measure prevalence and identified determinants of cannabinoid prescriptions for the management of chronic noncancer pain among physicians	166 physicians (family physicians/GPs and other specialties) answered a questionnaire (response rate of 52.2%)	Experiences: 27% had prescribed cannabinoids for all potential indications in the previous year. 23% had prescribed it for chronic noncancer pain, and of these 18% were medical cannabis. The majority had prescribed it to less than five patients. Physicians were not comfortable prescribing cannabinoids, with about 80% reporting a degree of comfort below 6 on a 1–10-point scale. Physicians reported medical education and having guidelines and more clinical data as factors which could increase their comfort level. Low level of comfort with prescribing medical cannabis for chronic noncancer pain was associated with low prevalence of prescription (OR: 1.25, CI: 1,01–1,55)	See the chapter "Procedures and definitions of medical cannabis prescriptions in included studies"

(continued)

(continued)

Reference	Country	Objective	Study population and methods	Results/conclusion	Comments
Ziemianski et al. (2015)	Canada	To determine physicians' educational needs regarding medical cannabis	426 physicians (44% GPs/family physicians and 51% other specialists, 4% other) answered a questionnaire (response rate: 1%, calculated from reported numbers)	Experiences: 79% had been approached by a patient to discuss the use of medical cannabis, and 39% had initiated a discussion with the patient about it. 59% had ever prescribed medical cannabis. There was a gap between current and desired knowledge concerning dosing, development and treatment plans, and the physicians reported a need for better knowledge of risks and benefits Attitudes and beliefs: 65% were concerned that patients who requested medical cannabis actually wanted it for recreational purposes. The majority of physicians reported that no other health professionals than physicians should be authorised to approve medical cannabis	See the chapter "procedures and definitions of medical cannabis prescriptions in included studies"

(continued)

(continued)

Reference	Country	Objective	Study population and methods	Results/conclusion	Comments
Fitzcharles et al. (2014)	Canada	To examine confidence in the knowledge of cannabinoids among rheumatologists	128 rheumatologists answered a questionnaire (response rate: 25%) The study compared responders who are confident and not confident in knowledge of cannabinoids	Experiences: 13% had ever recommended medical cannabis, and 90% were not confident in writing a prescription when required to indicate dosing, frequency, and method of administration. The study found that 7% of the not-confident versus 27% of the confident rheumatologists had previously recommended a trial of medical cannabis ($p = 0.006$) Attitudes and beliefs: 25% believed there was a role for medical cannabis in the management of rheumatic diseases. Barriers which would prevent physicians from prescribing medical cannabis were history/potential of drug abuse/addiction, mental health and lack of clear diagnosis/non-severity of pain complaints. 42% of the confident physicians would prescribe medical cannabis if all conventional treatments had failed, which only 23% of the non-confident physicians would	See the chapter "procedures and definitions of medical cannabis prescriptions in included studies"

(continued)

(continued)

Reference	Country	Objective	Study population and methods	Results/conclusion	Comments
Crowley et al. (2017)	Ireland	To assess levels of support for use of medical cannabis among GPs	565 GPs answered a questionnaire (response rate 15%) The study compares GPs with and without special training in addiction treatment	Attitudes and beliefs: almost 60% supported legislation of cannabis for medical use. GPs with training in addiction treatment were significantly less supportive that cannabis should be legalised for medical use compares to GPs with no training [65.1% vs. 78.5% respectively ($p = 0.003$)] GPs with training in addiction treatment were significantly less supportive that medical cannabis has a role in pain management (80.1% vs. 88.2%, $p = 0.03$), treatment of multiple sclerosis (85.5 vs. 92.4%, $p = 0.04$), and palliative care (83.3% vs. 90.0%, $p = 0.05$), compared to GPs with no training	See the chapter "procedures and definitions of medical cannabis prescriptions in included studies"
Van Hout et al. (2017)	Ireland	To study levels of support for medical cannabis among GPs	565 GPs answered a qualitative survey with open-ended questions (response rate: 15%)	Attitudes and beliefs: the identified attitudes were mixed and centred on the evidence base and quality control. Some physicians were convinced about effects but concerned about the lack of evidence and patient misuse	See the chapter "procedures and definitions of medical cannabis prescriptions in included studies"

(continued)

(continued)

Reference	Country	Objective	Study population and methods	Results/conclusion	Comments
Sharon et al. (2018)	Israel	To examine the attitudes, beliefs, and personal experience of pain specialists (physicians) in Israel regarding the medical use of cannabis	50 registered, active, board-certified pain specialists answered a web-based questionnaire (response rate: 64%)	Experiences: 64% of all practicing pain specialists in Israel responded. 95% of them prescribed medical cannabis. Among them, 63% found cannabis moderately to highly effective, 56% have encountered mild or no side effects, and only 5% perceived it as significantly harmful. Common indications were neuropathic pain (65%), oncological pain (50%), arthralgias (25%), and any intractable pain (29%). Leading contraindications were schizophrenia (76%), pregnancy/breastfeeding (65%), and age < 18 years (59%) Attitudes and beliefs: only 12% rated medical cannabis as more hazardous than opiates. 54% would like to see cannabis legalized in Israel. The majority (80%) reported they were inadequately trained to prescribe medical cannabis	See the chapter "procedures and definitions of medical cannabis prescriptions in included studies"

(continued)

(continued)

Reference	Country	Objective	Study population and methods	Results/conclusion	Comments
Zolotov et al. (2018)	Israel	To study physicians' views of medical cannabis and its possible integration into clinical practice	Qualitative interviews with 24 physicians (specialists or physicians currently specializing in oncology, pain medicine, and family medicine) were conducted	Attitudes and beliefs: The study identified two major narratives: (1) Cannabis as non-medicine: Conventional medicine was seen as the ideal option and physicians pointed out that medical cannabis failed to comply with the standards of biomedicine. Physicians pointed out the lack of scientific evidence of safety and efficacy. They presented medical cannabis as a social and criminal matter, which should not fall under the professional domain of medicine (2) Cannabis as medicine: Hands-on experience was mentioned as having a crucial impact on attitudes and practices. Physicians pointed out the limitations of evidence-based medicine and argued that other aspects of health care are unsupported by evidence. When considering very sick people, physicians gave much less weight to the lack of evidence and potential harms. Besides, cannabis was described as medicine for patients with an uncontested diagnosis which can be proved by objective laboratory procedures	See the chapter "procedures and definitions of medical cannabis prescriptions in included studies"

(continued)

(continued)

Reference	Country	Objective	Study population and methods	Results/conclusion	Comments
Ablin et al. (2016)	Israel	To survey rheumatologists' attitudes towards the use of medical cannabis	23 rheumatologists answered a questionnaire (response rate of 19.3%)	Experiences: 48% had previously prescribed medical cannabis, and 78% were not confident in writing prescriptions when required to indicate dosing, frequency and method of administration Attitudes and beliefs: 83% were willing to prescribe medical cannabis if conventional treatments failed, and 9% would prescribe it regardless of previous treatments	See the chapter "procedures and definitions of medical cannabis prescriptions in included studies"

(continued)

(continued)

Reference	Country	Objective	Study population and methods	Results/conclusion	Comments
Ebert et al. (2015)	Israel	To examine physicians' experiences, knowledge and attitudes towards medical cannabis	27 physicians (various specialities: oncology, pain medicine, rehabilitation, psychiatry and neurology) answered a questionnaire (response rate of 72%) The study compared physicians who had ever recommended medical cannabis with those who had not	Experiences: about 90% have been exposed to a patient using medical cannabis, and 60% had recommended it to at least one patient. Compared to physicians who had never recommended medical cannabis (40.3%), physicians who had recommended it once or more (59.7) reported themselves as having a significantly greater knowledge of dosage, ways of administration and risk and adverse effects ($p < 0.05$) Clinical experiences and knowledge from medical literature and other physicians were influencing physicians' decision on recommendation of medical cannabis Attitudes and beliefs: about 80% reported that medical cannabis could be helpful for chronically and terminally ill patients. About 60% reported that physicians should not be permitted to prescribe it to patients directly, without the Ministry of Health's licensing procedure. 88% reported a need for more education on medical cannabis	See the chapter "procedures and definitions of medical cannabis prescriptions in included studies"

Source Rønne et al. (2021, pp. 6–18)

References

Ablin, J., Ste-Marie, P. A., Schäfer, M., Häuser, W., & Fitzcharles, M. A. (2016). Medical use of cannabis products: Lessons to be learned from Israel and Canada. *Schmerz (Berlin, Germany)*, *30*(1), 3–13. https://doi.org/10.1007/s00482-015-0083-4

Bega, D., Simuni, T., Okun, M. S., Chen, X., & Schmidt, P. (2017). Medicinal cannabis for Parkinson's disease: practices, beliefs, and attitudes among providers at National Parkinson Foundation Centers of Excellence. *Movement Disorders Clinical Practice*, *4*(1), 90–95. https://doi.org/10.1002/mdc3.12359

Braun, I. M., Wright, A., Peteet, J., Meyer, F. L., Yuppa, D. P., Bolcic-Jankovic, D., … & Campbell, E. G. (2018). Medical oncologists' beliefs, practices, and knowledge regarding marijuana used therapeutically: A nationally representative survey study. *Journal of Clinical Oncology*, *36*(19), 1957. https://doi.org/10.1200/JCO.2017.76.1221

Charuvastra, A., Friedmann, P. D., & Stein, M. D. (2005). Physician attitudes regarding the prescription of medical marijuana. *Journal of Addictive Diseases*, *24*(3), 87–93. https://doi.org/10.1300/J069v24n03_07

Crowley, D., Collins, C., Delargy, I., Laird, E., & Van Hout, M. C. (2017). Irish general practitioner attitudes toward decriminalisation and medical use of cannabis: Results from a national survey. *Harm Reduction Journal*, *14*, 1–8. https://doi.org/10.1186/s12954-016-0129-7

Ebert, T., Zolotov, Y., Eliav, S., Ginzburg, O., Shapira, I., & Magnezi, R. (2015). Assessment of Israeli physicians' knowledge, experience and attitudes towards medical cannabis: A pilot study. *The Israel Medical Association Journal: IMAJ*, *17*(7), 437–441.

Fitzcharles, M. A., Ste-Marie, P. A., Clauw, D. J., Jamal, S., Karsh, J., LeClercq, S., … & Walsh, Z. (2014). Rheumatologists lack confidence in their knowledge of cannabinoids pertaining to the management of rheumatic complaints. *BMC Musculoskeletal Disorders*, *15*(1), 1–6. https://doi.org/10.1186/1471-2474-15-258

Irvine, G. (2006). Rural doctors' attitudes to and knowledge of medicinal cannabis. *Journal of Law and Medicine*, *14*(1), 135–142.

Jacobs, N. I., Montebello, M., Monds, L. A., & Lintzeris, N. (2019). Survey of Australian psychiatrists' and psychiatry trainees' knowledge about and attitudes towards medicinal cannabinoids. *Australasian Psychiatry: Bulletin of Royal Australian and New Zealand College of Psychiatrists*, *27*(1), 80–85. https://doi.org/10.1177/1039856218803675

Karanges, E. A., Suraev, A., Elias, N., Manocha, R., & McGregor, I. S. (2018). Knowledge and attitudes of Australian general practitioners towards medicinal cannabis: a cross-sectional survey. *BMJ Open*, *8*(7), e022101. https://doi.org/10.1136/bmjopen-2018-022101

Kondrad, E., & Reid, A. (2013). Colorado family physicians' attitudes toward medical marijuana. *The Journal of the American Board of Family Medicine*, *26*(1), 52–60. https://doi.org/10.3122/jabfm.2013.01.120089

Luba, R., Earleywine, M., Farmer, S., & Slavin, M. (2018). Cannabis in end-of-life care: Examining attitudes and practices of palliative care providers. *Journal of Psychoactive Drugs*, *50*(4), 348–354. https://doi.org/10.1080/02791072.2018.1462543

Mathern, G. W., Beninsig, L., & Nehlig, A. (2015). Fewer specialists support using medical marijuana and CBD in treating epilepsy patients compared with other medical professionals and patients: Result of Epilepsia's survey. *Epilepsia*, *56*(1), 1–6. https://doi.org/10.1111/epi.12843

Philpot, L. M., Ebbert, J. O., & Hurt, R. T. (2019). A survey of the attitudes, beliefs and knowledge about medical cannabis among primary care providers. *BMC Family Practice*, *20*, 1–7. https://doi.org/10.1186/s12875-019-0906-y

Robinson, E., Murphy, E., & Friedman, A. (2018). Knowledge, attitudes, and perceptions of cannabinoids in the dermatology community. *Journal of Drugs in Dermatology: JDD*, *17*(12), 1273–1278.

Rønne, S. T., Rosenbaek, F., Pedersen, L. B., Waldorff, F. B., Nielsen, J. B., Riisgaard, H., & Søndergaard, J. (2021). Physicians' experiences, attitudes, and beliefs towards medical cannabis: A systematic literature review. *BMC Family Practice*, *22*(1), 212. https://doi.org/10.1186/s12875-021-01559-w

Sharon, H., Goldway, N., Goor-Aryeh, I., Eisenberg, E., & Brill, S. (2018). Personal experience and attitudes of pain medicine specialists in Israel regarding the medical use of cannabis for chronic pain. *Journal of Pain Research*, 1411–1419. https://doi.org/10.2147/JPR.S159852

Sideris, A., Khan, F., Boltunova, A., Cuff, G., Gharibo, C., & Doan, L. V. (2018). New York physicians' perspectives and knowledge of the state medical marijuana program. *Cannabis and Cannabinoid Research*, *3*(1), 74–84. https://doi.org/10.1089/can.2017.0046

St-Amant, H., Ware, M. A., Julien, N., & Lacasse, A. (2015). Prevalence and determinants of cannabinoid prescription for the management of chronic noncancer pain: A postal survey of physicians in the Abitibi-Témiscamingue region of Quebec. *Canadian Medical Association Open Access Journal*, *3*(2), E251–E257. https://doi.org/10.9778/cmajo.20140095

Van Hout, M. C., Collins, C., Delargy, I., & Crowley, D. (2017). Irish general practitioner (GP) perspectives toward decriminalisation, legalisation and cannabis for therapeutic purposes (CTP). *International Journal of Mental Health and Addiction*, *15*, 670–683. https://doi.org/10.1007/s11469-016-9710-2

Ziemianski, D., Capler, R., Tekanoff, R., Lacasse, A., Luconi, F., & Ware, M. A. (2015). Cannabis in medicine: A national educational needs assessment among Canadian physicians. *BMC Medical Education*, *15*(1), 1–7. https://doi.org/10.1186/s12909-015-0335-0

Zolotov, Y., Vulfsons, S., Zarhin, D., & Sznitman, S. (2018). Medical cannabis: An oxymoron? Physicians' perceptions of medical cannabis. *International Journal of Drug Policy*, *57*, 4–10. https://doi.org/10.1016/j.drugpo.2018.03.025

Appendix F
Studies in Cheng et al.'s (2022) Article

See Tables F.1 and F.2.

Table F.1 Studies included in this review about chronic noncancer pain

Author (year), country	Aims	Study design	Sample	Study findings
Ablin et al. (2016), Israel	Achieve a cross-cultural comparison with Canada on rheumatologists' confidence of knowledge of MC	Survey from Fitzcharles et al. (2014) study	$N = 23$ rheumatology specialists and residents	78% rheumatologists were not confident in writing prescriptions for MC, 48% believed in its therapeutic role for rheumatic diseases, 51% have previously prescribed it. MC would be considered if patients were refractory to conventional treatment by 82.6%
Abo Ziad et al. (2020), Israel	Assess the attitudes and beliefs of Israeli family physicians on the use of MC and their knowledge on adverse effects and barriers to use	Survey	$N = 152$ physicians (97 specialists, 48 residents, three general practitioners)	High proportions of family physicians believed MC is effective in cancer pain (84.2%) and chronic pain (82.2%). They generally believed specialists in pain medicine and oncology should recommend it. They themselves were *not willing* to prescribe or only *willing to a small extent*

(continued)

G. Bennett, *A Scoping Review of Clinical Studies About the Therapeutic Benefits of Medical Cannabis*, https://doi.org/10.1007/978-981-97-7941-3

Table F.1 (continued)

Author (year), country	Aims	Study design	Sample	Study findings
Amfinsen et al. (2021), Norway	Assess Norwegian physicians' perceived knowledge of, experience with, and attitudes toward MC	Survey	$N = 102$ physicians	Of the physicians who were asked to choose justifications for why MC should be available by prescription in Norway, the majority stated that MC can improve the quality of life for patients with chronic pain and MC may reduce unnecessary use of opioids
Bega et al. (2017), International	Assess MC-related practices, experiences, beliefs, and attitudes of neurologists across National Parkinson's Foundation Center of Excellence	Survey	$N = 56$ neurologists	Physicians described a lack of formal education on MC, reported obtaining their information from medical literature and personal experience, and wanted more attention to MC in the curricula. Concerning side effects noted include negative impact on memory, executive function, driving, and addiction
Carlini et al. (2015), USA	Assess Washington State's healthcare providers' MC knowledge, beliefs, clinical practices, and training needs	Survey	$N = 494$ healthcare providers (physicians, physician assistants, nurses, pharmacists)	Intractable pain was the leading indication for written authorizations. Despite healthcare providers' eligibility to write MC authorizations, the majority has not issued one. There was general support for formal training and concerns for addiction and psychiatric side effects

(continued)

Table F.1 (continued)

Author (year), country	Aims	Study design	Sample	Study findings
Collister et al. (2021), Canada	Elicit Canadian nephrologists' views regarding the use and study of MC in patients with kidney disease	Survey	$N = 154$ nephrologists	Chronic pain was one of the major indications for a MC prescription but only 19% of nephrologists have prescribed MC for it. Greater support for MC use in chronic pain if symptoms were refractory to or patients could not tolerate conventional treatment. However, nephrologists did not feel comfortable prescribing MC themselves and preferred someone else do it with more prescribing expertise and a license. Concerns expressed include the lack of evidence for safety and efficacy and uncertainty with dosing
Cooke et al. (2019), USA	Present patients' and clinicians' perspectives on the co-use of MC and opioid among chronic noncancer pain patients with a history of a substance-use disorder and their clinicians	Semistructured interviews	$N = 23$ primary care providers (18 physicians, four nurse practitioners, one physician assistant)	Clinicians did not routinely discuss MC with patients, but noted that MC was helpful to their patients in managing pain symptoms while on opioids. Clinicians were not comfortable to discuss and/or provide MC in clinical settings and expressed concerns about potential exacerbation of mental health issues with MC use

(continued)

Table F.1 (continued)

Author (year), country	Aims	Study design	Sample	Study findings
Crowley et al. (2017), Ireland	Investigate attitudes of Irish general practitioners (GPs) attitudes toward decriminalization of MC and assess levels of support for use of MC	Survey	$N = 565$ GPs	> 60% Irish GPs agreed that MC has a role in pain management and 58.6% supported legalization for medical use. Support for legalization was higher in those who were trained in addiction treatment (e.g., managing opioid users). Majority of Irish GPs did not support decriminalization of MC for recreational use but GPs with more advanced addiction specialist training supported decriminalization of MC
Ebert et al. (2015), Israel	Examine the experience, knowledge, and attitudes of Israeli physicians of different specialties toward MC, and assess whether physicians with more knowledge or experience have different attitudes than those who are less knowledgeable and experienced	Survey	$N = 72$ physicians (28 oncology, five pain, 20 psychiatry, 13 neurology, six rehabilitation)	Pain was two of the four most prevalent indications for MC use (chronic pain, cancer pain, chemotherapy-induced symptoms, palliative care). Oncologists and pain physicians generally disagreed that MC undermined mental health. Physicians who recommended MC reported themselves having greater knowledge. Physicians unanimously agreed that more education on MC should be available to physicians and specific training should precede ability to recommend MC

(continued)

Table F.1 (continued)

Author (year), country	Aims	Study design	Sample	Study findings
Fitzcharles et al. (2014), Canada	Examine rheumatologists' confidence about cannabinoids in general and their ability to advise patients about MC	Survey	$N = 128$ rheumatologists	45% rheumatologists believed there is no therapeutic role for MC in the management of rheumatic diseases, 70% have never previously recommended any form of MC for patients and 60% currently would not recommend a trial of any MC
Irvine et al. (2006), Australia	Obtain information about GPs' views on potential legalization of MC	Survey	$N = 32$ GPs	GPs generally regarded chronic pain as a MC-treatable condition. They would prescribe MC if it was legal, backed up by research, and under a legalized regulatory scheme for indications. There was concern of bureaucracy of paperwork with the public knowing about MC access
Jacobs et al. (2019), Australia	Assess Australia psychiatrists' and psychiatry trainees' knowledge, attitudes, and concerns about MC	Survey	$N = 23$ psychiatrists	> 2/3 respondents believed there was evidence for use of CBD and THC in treating chronic pain. They generally could not differentiate between CBD and THC indications. 55% were open to prescribing MC if it were legal. Greatest concerns regarded psychotic symptoms, recreational use (for intoxication), apathy, addiction, and dependence

(continued)

Table F.1 (continued)

Author (year), country	Aims	Study design	Sample	Study findings
Karanges et al. (2018), Australia	Examine the knowledge and attitudes of Australian GPs toward MC	Survey	$N = 640$ GPs	61.5% GPs have fielded at least one enquiry about MC in the last 3 months, but half were not comfortable dealing with enquiries. They believed in the utility of MC, but generally did not want to prescribe MC, citing risk of abuse and dependence as primary concerns. GPs preferred training and accreditation or a shared care arrangement with a specialist instead of a specialist-only prescribing approach. Most rated themselves having poor perceived knowledge of MC. There was a contrast in support for MC for patients with chronic cancer pain (80.2%) and chronic noncancer pain (39.1%)
Kondrad and Reid (2013), USA	Gather information about Colorado family physicians' experience with and attitudes toward MC	Survey	$N = 520$ family physicians	Despite Colorado having the highest per-capita number of patients using MC, 31% of family physicians never recommended MC. Most physicians did not think there are significant health benefits to MC. Those who have not recommended MC before cited news media, practice policy, personal opinion, concerns of legal liability, and a lack of evidence as influencing factors. Physicians believed MC is predominantly used by people who want legal protection for recreational cannabis. They expressed a strong desire for educational opportunities

(continued)

Table F.1 (continued)

Author (year), country	Aims	Study design	Sample	Study findings
Mitchell et al. (2016), Canada	Determine hospital pharmacists' opinions about MC and their level of comfort in providing advice about MC to patients and other healthcare professionals	Survey	$N = 769$ hospital pharmacists	Majority obtained self-directed education on MC. Despite limited education, 53.8% of hospital pharmacists have been confronted with questions about its use. 67% disagreed that they were knowledgeable about MC, and 50% completely disagreed that they were comfortable in providing advice to patients
Narouze et al. (2020), USA	Characterize pain physicians' advocacy and concerns regarding MC	Survey	$N = 30$ pain physicians	Pain physicians believed in the legitimacy and benefits of MC for physical symptoms and 76% have cared for patients on MC. However, 13% participants were actually registered in an MC program
Philpot et al. (2019), USA	Understand the attitudes, beliefs, and knowledge of primary care providers and identify ongoing barriers, biases, and knowledge gaps relating to MC	Survey	$N = 62$ primary care providers (physicians, nurse practitioners, physician assistants)	Providers believed that MC is a legitimate medical therapy for intractable pain but did not believe it can improve patient's quality of life. One third were concerned about significant drug interactions with MC. 50% were not ready or did not want to answer patient questions regarding MC

(continued)

Table F.1 (continued)

Author (year), country	Aims	Study design	Sample	Study findings
Sharon et al. (2018), Israel	Examine the attitudes, beliefs, and personal experiences of Israeli pain specialists regarding the MC	Survey	$N = 50$ pain specialists	95% prescribed MC in their pain practice, 63% found it moderately to highly effective in treating patients with intractable chronic pain, 81% felt that they have not received adequate education regarding MC during their specialty training. There was general agreement that MC has a favorable side effect profile compared to opiates yet most preferred trialing opiate therapy before initiating MC. Doctors favored chronic pain states with a clear etiology and viewed psychiatric morbidity, breastfeeding, and young age to be leading contraindications. Most physicians overestimated addiction rates
Sideris et al. (2018), USA	Assess New York's physicians' comfort level, opinions, and experience in recommending or supporting patient use of MC	Survey	$N = 164$ physicians (primary care, anesthesiology, pain medicine, surgery, psychiatry)	87% respondents were not registered with New York's MC program, but majority were willing to recommend patients to registered physicians. Pain symptom control was the most common symptom qualifying for MC. ~ 75% opioid prescribers considered recommending MC as an adjuvant in pain

(continued)

Table F.1 (continued)

Author (year), country	Aims	Study design	Sample	Study findings
Starrels et al. (2020), USA	Generate consensus among clinicians expert in chronic pain and opioid prescribing about how to respond to MC use among patients on long-term opioid therapy (LTOT)	Analysis from an online Delphi study	$N = 42$ clinicians (physicians, nurse practitioners, clinical pharmacologist, registered nurse, clinical nurse specialist)	There was expert consensus about initiating monitoring strategies in response to MC use among patients prescribed LTOT; tapering or discontinuation of LTOT was not important for one-time or occasional MC users. There was disagreement as to whether to taper or discontinue opioids for patients with a pattern of repeated use and a suspicion of a cannabis use disorder

Source Cheng et al. (2022, pp. 722–725)

Table F.2 Studies included in this review about chronic cancer pain

Author (year), country	Aims	Study design	Sample	Study findings
Braun et al. (2017), U.S.A.	Investigate the extent to which oncology experts view marijuana as having medical value and the range of approaches to clinical decision making around MC	Semistructured interviews	$N = 15$ oncology experts (10 oncologists, two palliative care physicians, one psychiatrist, one surgeon)	13 of 15 of oncology experts endorsed MC for the indication of pain. Expert opinion was divided on MC's position in medicine with about half who believed MC to have efficacy comparable to conventional management strategies. Nearly as many viewed it as an adjunct, capable of reducing benzodiazepine and opioid loads

(continued)

Table F.2 (continued)

Author (year), country	Aims	Study design	Sample	Study findings
Braun et al. (2018), U.S.A.	Examine beliefs, knowledge, and practices of oncologists regarding MC	Survey	$N = 237$ oncologists	There was a lack of consensus among oncologists regarding MC as the primary treatment for pain, but > 2/3 supported its use as an adjunct to standard pain management strategies. 45.9% reported discussing about MC with patients in the past year, 56.7% of them did not consider themselves sufficiently knowledgeable to make MC recommendations
Luba et al. (2018), U.S.A.	Examine the attitudes, beliefs, and practices of palliative and hospice care providers regarding the use of MC for terminally ill patients	Survey	$N = 426$ palliative and hospice care providers (345 doctors, 58 nurses)	Majority of palliative and hospice care providers saw MC as helpful in treating pain and end of life generally, and useful as an adjuvant medicine. However, fewer than half (46.4%) have recommended MC in the past. 61% indicated that they would recommend MC for terminal illness regardless of legality
Uritsky et al. (2011), U.S.A.	Assess the knowledge, experience, and views of hospice professionals regarding the use of MC in terminally ill patients	Survey	$N = 209$ hospice professionals (13 medical doctors, 131 nurses, 34 social workers)	90% hospice care professionals supported the legalization of MC for palliative symptoms. Pain control was the most commonly perceived reason for marijuana use though not a currently FDA-approved indication. Majority would neglect ethical implications with smoking MC if it was controlling symptoms

(continued)

Table F.2 (continued)

Author (year), country	Aims	Study design	Sample	Study findings
Zolotov et al. (2018), Israel	Understand the views of physicians who regularly encounter cancer and chronic pain patients on MC and its possible integration into their clinic, and identify potential underlying factors that influence these perceptions	Semiconstructed interviews	*N* = 24 physicians (six pain medicine, nine oncology, nine family medicine)	On one hand, physicians abiding by the evidence-base paradigm of healthcare did not see MC as a conventional medicine. Some physicians viewed patients as drug addicts and feared recreational use of medically acquired cannabis. On the other hand, physicians saw MC as a viable treatment for pain and suffering especially for cancer patients
Zolotov et al. (2019), Israel	Identify underlying factors that influence physicians' intentions to recommend MC to patients	Survey and some interviews	*N* = 247 physicians (98 family physicians, 80 oncologists, 69 pain medicine)	Respondents had higher intentions to recommend MC to the cancer patient than the chronic pain patient. There were more psychosocial (nonmedical) factors associated with intentions to recommend MC to the chronic pain patient

Source Cheng et al. (2022, p. 726)

References

Ablin, J. N., Elkayam, O., & Fitzcharles, M. A. (2016). Attitudes of Israeli rheumatologists to the use of medical cannabis as therapy for rheumatic disorders. *Rambam Maimonides Medical Journal*, *7*(2). https://doi.org/10.5041/RMMJ.10239

Abo Ziad, R., Grynbaum, M. B., Peleg, R., & Treister-Goltzman, Y. (2022). The attitudes and beliefs of family physicians regarding the use of medical cannabis, knowledge of side effects, and barriers to use: a comparison between residents and specialists. *American Journal of Therapeutics*, *29*(4), e400–e409. https://doi.org/10.1097/MJT.0000000000001236

Arnfinsen, J. L., & Kisa, A. (2021). Assessment of Norwegian physicians' knowledge, experience and attitudes towards medical cannabis. *Drugs: Education, Prevention and Policy*, *28*(2), 165–171. https://doi.org/10.1080/09687637.2020.1806208

Bega, D., Simuni, T., Okun, M. S., Chen, X., & Schmidt, P. (2016). Medicinal cannabis for Parkinson's disease: Practices, beliefs, and attitudes among providers at national Parkinson foundation centers of excellence. *Movement Disorders Clinical Practice*, *4*(1), 90–95. https://doi.org/10.1002/mdc3.12359

Braun, I. M., Meyer, F. L., Gagne, J. J., Nabati, L., Yuppa, D. P., Carmona, M. A., Burstein, H. J., Suzuki, J., Nayak, M. M., & Martins, Y. (2017). Experts' perspectives on the role of medical marijuana in oncology: A semistructured interview study. *Psycho-oncology*, *26*(8), 1087–1092. https://doi.org/10.1002/pon.4365

Braun, I. M., Wright, A., Peteet, J., Meyer, F. L., Yuppa, D. P., Bolcic-Jankovic, D., LeBlanc, J., Chang, Y., Yu, L., Nayak, M. M., Tulsky, J. A., Suzuki, J., Nabati, L., & Campbell, E. G. (2018). Medical oncologists' beliefs, practices, and knowledge regarding marijuana used therapeutically: A nationally representative survey study. *Journal of Clinical Oncology: Official Journal of the American Society of Clinical Oncology*, *36*(19), 1957–1962. https://doi.org/10.1200/JCO.2017.76.1221

Carlini, B. H., Garrett, S. B., & Carter, G. T. (2017). Medicinal cannabis: A survey among health care providers in Washington State. *American Journal of Hospice and Palliative Medicine®*, *34*(1), 85–91. https://doi.org/10.1177/1049909115604669

Cheng, K. Y. C., Harnett, J. E., Davis, S. R., Eassey, D., Law, S., & Smith, L. (2022). Health-care professionals' perspectives on the use of medicinal cannabis to manage chronic pain: A systematic search and narrative review. *Pain Practice: The Official Journal of World Institute of Pain*, *22*(8), 718–732. https://doi.org/10.1111/papr.13161

Collister, D., Tennankore, K., Davison, S. N., Wald, R., Rabbat, C., & Walsh, M. (2021). Nephrologist views regarding cannabinoid use in advanced chronic kidney disease and dialysis: A survey. *Journal of Pain and Symptom Management*, *61*(2), 237–245.e2. https://doi.org/10.1016/j.jpainsymman.2020.08.003

Cooke, A. C., Knight, K. R., & Miaskowski, C. (2019). Patients' and clinicians' perspectives of co-use of cannabis and opioids for chronic non-cancer pain management in primary care. *The International Journal on Drug Policy*, *63*, 23–28. https://doi.org/10.1016/j.drugpo.2018.09.002

Crowley, D., Collins, C., Delargy, I., Laird, E., & Van Hout, M. C. (2017). Irish general practitioner attitudes toward decriminalisation and medical use of cannabis: Results from a national survey. *Harm Reduction Journal*, *14*(1), 4. https://doi.org/10.1186/s12954-016-0129-7

Ebert, T., Zolotov, Y., Eliav, S., Ginzburg, O., Shapira, I., & Magnezi, R. (2015). Assessment of Israeli physicians' knowledge, experience and attitudes towards medical cannabis: A pilot study. *The Israel Medical Association Journal: IMAJ*, *17*(7), 437–441.

Fitzcharles, M. A., Ste-Marie, P. A., Clauw, D. J., Jamal, S., Karsh, J., LeClercq, S., McDougall, J. J., Shir, Y., Shojania, K., & Walsh, Z. (2014). Rheumatologists lack confidence in their knowledge of cannabinoids pertaining to the management of rheumatic complaints. *BMC Musculoskeletal Disorders*, *15*, 258. https://doi.org/10.1186/1471-2474-15-258

Irvine G. (2006). Rural doctors' attitudes to and knowledge of medicinal cannabis. *Journal of Law and Medicine*, *14*(1), 135–142.

Jacobs, N. I., Montebello, M., Monds, L. A., & Lintzeris, N. (2019). Survey of Australian psychiatrists' and psychiatry trainees' knowledge about and attitudes towards medicinal cannabinoids. *Australasian Psychiatry: Bulletin of Royal Australian and New Zealand College of Psychiatrists*, *27*(1), 80–85. https://doi.org/10.1177/1039856218803675

Karanges, E. A., Suraev, A., Elias, N., Manocha, R., & McGregor, I. S. (2018). Knowledge and attitudes of Australian general practitioners towards medicinal cannabis: A cross-sectional survey. *BMJ Open*, *8*(7), e022101. https://doi.org/10.1136/bmjopen-2018-022101

Kondrad, E., & Reid, A. (2013). Colorado family physicians' attitudes toward medical marijuana. *Journal of the American Board of Family Medicine: JABFM*, *26*(1), 52-60. https://doi.org/10.3122/jabfm.2013.01.120089

Luba, R., Earleywine, M., Farmer, S., & Slavin, M. (2018). Cannabis in end-of-life care: Examining attitudes and practices of palliative care providers. *Journal of Psychoactive Drugs*, *50*(4), 348–354. https://doi.org/10.1080/02791072.2018.1462543

Mitchell, F., Gould, O., LeBlanc, M., & Manuel, L. (2016). Opinions of hospital pharmacists in Canada regarding marijuana for medical purposes. *The Canadian Journal of Hospital Pharmacy*, *69*(2), 122–130. https://doi.org/10.4212/cjhp.v69i2.1539

Narouze, S., Hakim, S. M., Kohan, L., Adams, D., & Souza, D. (2020). Medical cannabis attitudes and beliefs among pain physicians. *Regional Anesthesia and Pain Medicine*, *45*(11), 917–919. https://doi.org/10.1136/rapm-2020-101658

Philpot, L. M., Ebbert, J. O., & Hurt, R. T. (2019). A survey of the attitudes, beliefs and knowledge about medical cannabis among primary care providers. *BMC Family Practice*, *20*(1), 17. https://doi.org/10.1186/s12875-019-0906-y

Sharon, H., Goldway, N., Goor-Aryeh, I., Eisenberg, E., & Brill, S. (2018). Personal experience and attitudes of pain medicine specialists in Israel regarding the medical use of cannabis for chronic pain. *Journal of Pain Research*, *11*, 1411–1419. https://doi.org/10.2147/JPR.S159852

Sideris, A., Khan, F., Boltunova, A., Cuff, G., Gharibo, C., & Doan, L. V. (2018). New York physicians' perspectives and knowledge of the state medical Marijuana Program. *Cannabis and Cannabinoid Research*, *3*(1), 74–84. https://doi.org/10.1089/can.2017.0046

Starrels, J. L., Young, S. R., Azari, S. S., Becker, W. C., Jennifer Edelman, E., Liebschutz, J. M., Pomeranz, J., Roy, P., Saini, S., & Merlin, J. S. (2020). Disagreement and uncertainty among experts about how to respond to marijuana use in patients on long-term opioids for chronic pain: Results of a Delphi Study. *Pain medicine (Malden, Mass.)*, *21*(2), 247–254. https://doi.org/10.1093/pm/pnz153

Uritsky, T. J., McPherson, M. L., & Pradel, F. (2011). Assessment of hospice health professionals' knowledge, views, and experience with medical marijuana. *Journal of Palliative Medicine*, *14*(12), 1291–1295. https://doi.org/10.1089/jpm.2011.0113

Zolotov, Y., Vulfsons, S., & Sznitman, S. (2019). Predicting physicians' intentions to recommend medical cannabis. *Journal of Pain and Symptom Management*, *58*(3), 400–407. https://doi.org/10.1016/j.jpainsymman.2019.05.010

Zolotov, Y., Vulfsons, S., Zarhin, D., & Sznitman, S. (2018). Medical cannabis: An oxymoron? Physicians' perceptions of medical cannabis. *The International Journal on Drug Policy*, *57*, 4–10. https://doi.org/10.1016/j.drugpo.2018.03.025

The manufacturer's authorised representative in the EU is Springer
Nature Customer Service Centre GmbH, Europaplatz 3, 69115 Heidelberg,
Germany. If you have any concerns regarding our products, please
contact ProductSafety@springernature.com

Printed and bound by CPI Group (UK) Ltd, Croydon, CR0 4YY
01/10/2026
02225914-0003